CARDIO TRACKER

Equipment	Level	Duration	Calories	Equipment	Level	Duration	Calories

I0408202

BRAIN WAVES

ADJUSTMENTS

Equipment	Your Settings

Exercise	Sets	Exercise	Sets	Exercise	Sets

Exercise	Sets	Exercise	Sets	Exercise	Sets

Exercise	Sets	Exercise	Sets	Exercise	Sets

Exercise	Sets	Exercise	Sets	Exercise	Sets

Exercise	Sets	Exercise	Sets	Exercise	Sets

Exercise	Sets	Exercise	Sets	Exercise	Sets

Left, Right - Either or....!

Place a tick on any area you think requires some attention. Return in 3 weeks and decide if you need another tick and some more work on that area.

Remember your own observation may be "determined" by your thoughts of perfection. Looking at yourself from various angles can be misleading.

Don't be afraid to ask a colleague or your partner what they think...!

Isolated movements can bring on lagging muscles... Think about this when creating your next routine.

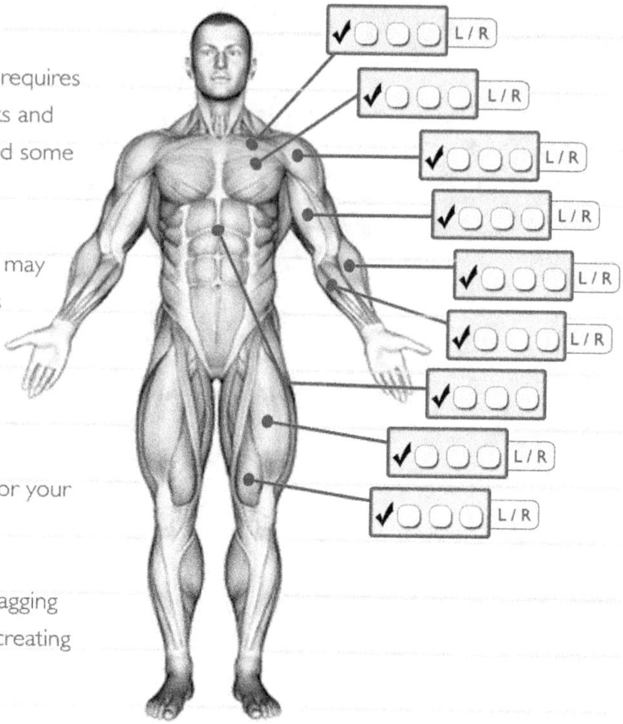

L / R
L / R
L / R
L / R
L / R
L / R
L / R
L / R

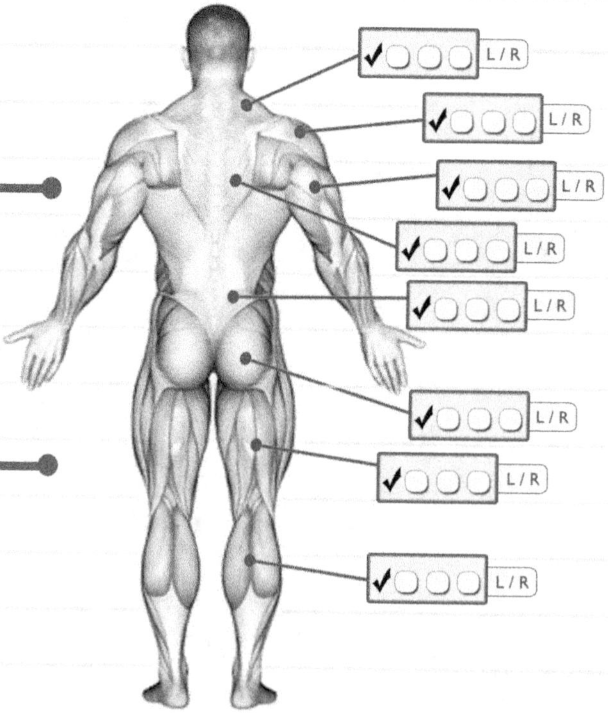

Date ☑
Date ☑
Date ☑
Date ☑

L / R
L / R
L / R
L / R
L / R
L / R
L / R
L / R

Before Your Journal - After Your Journal

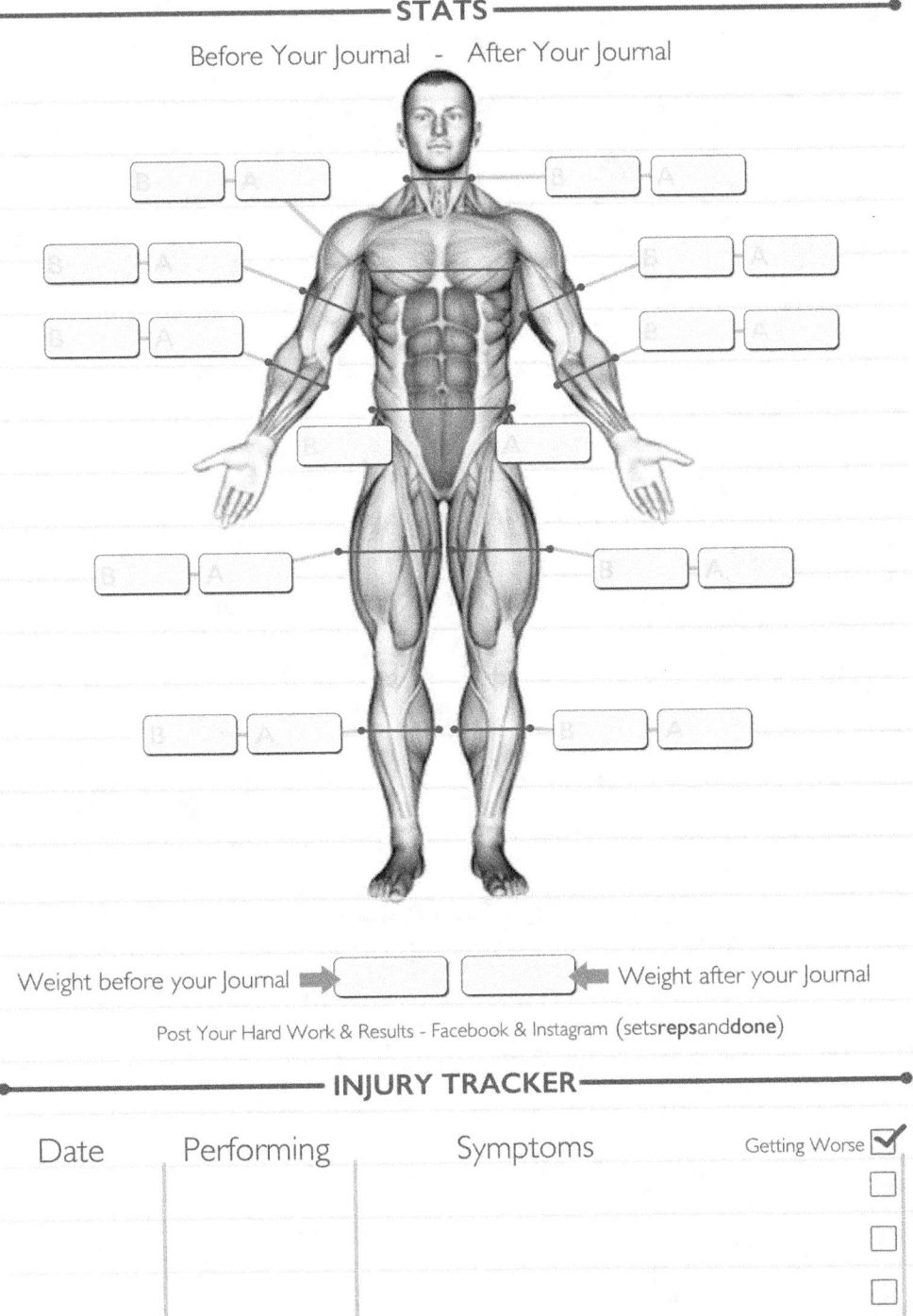

Weight before your Journal ➡️ [ ] [ ] ⬅️ Weight after your Journal

Post Your Hard Work & Results - Facebook & Instagram (**sets**reps**and**done)

INJURY TRACKER

Date	Performing	Symptoms	Getting Worse ☑️
			☐
			☐
			☐
			☐
			☐
			☐

Exercise	Weight	Date - Increase / Results					
		DATE		DATE		DATE	

PROTEIN TRACKER

	WEEKS 1,2,3,4		DAILY TARGET			

MEALS	•——1	•——2	•——3	•——4	•——5	•——6	DAILY TOTAL
MONDAY							
TUESDAY							
WEDNESDAY							
THURSDAY							
FRIDAY							
SATURDAY							
SUNDAY							
MONDAY							
TUESDAY							
WEDNESDAY							
THURSDAY							
FRIDAY							
SATURDAY							
SUNDAY							
MONDAY							
TUESDAY							
WEDNESDAY							
THURSDAY							
FRIDAY							
SATURDAY							
SUNDAY							
MONDAY							
TUESDAY							
WEDNESDAY							
THURSDAY							
FRIDAY							
SATURDAY							
SUNDAY							

PROTEIN TRACKER

WEEKS 5,6,7,8   DAILY TARGET [   ]

MEALS	•——1	•——2	•——3	•——4	•——5	•——6	DAILY TOTAL
MONDAY							
TUESDAY							
WEDNESDAY							
THURSDAY							
FRIDAY							
SATURDAY							
SUNDAY							
MONDAY							
TUESDAY							
WEDNESDAY							
THURSDAY							
FRIDAY							
SATURDAY							
SUNDAY							
MONDAY							
TUESDAY							
WEDNESDAY							
THURSDAY							
FRIDAY							
SATURDAY							
SUNDAY							
MONDAY							
TUESDAY							
WEDNESDAY							
THURSDAY							
FRIDAY							
SATURDAY							
SUNDAY							

PROTEIN TRACKER

WEEKS 9,10,11,12   DAILY TARGET [   ]

MEALS	•——1	•——2	•——3	•——4	•——5	•——6	DAILY TOTAL
MONDAY							
TUESDAY							
WEDNESDAY							
THURSDAY							
FRIDAY							
SATURDAY							
SUNDAY							
MONDAY							
TUESDAY							
WEDNESDAY							
THURSDAY							
FRIDAY							
SATURDAY							
SUNDAY							
MONDAY							
TUESDAY							
WEDNESDAY							
THURSDAY							
FRIDAY							
SATURDAY							
SUNDAY							
MONDAY							
TUESDAY							
WEDNESDAY							
THURSDAY							
FRIDAY							
SATURDAY							
SUNDAY							

EXERCISE	SETS	REPS AND DONE!			
		REPS ☐	REPS ☐	REPS ☐	REPS ☐
	WEIGHT				
		REPS ☐	REPS ☐	REPS ☐	REPS ☐
	WEIGHT				
		REPS ☐	REPS ☐	REPS ☐	REPS ☐
	WEIGHT				
		REPS ☐	REPS ☐	REPS ☐	REPS ☐
	WEIGHT				
		REPS ☐	REPS ☐	REPS ☐	REPS ☐
	WEIGHT				
		REPS ☐	REPS ☐	REPS ☐	REPS ☐
	WEIGHT				
		REPS ☐	REPS ☐	REPS ☐	REPS ☐
	WEIGHT				
		REPS ☐	REPS ☐	REPS ☐	REPS ☐
	WEIGHT				
		REPS ☐	REPS ☐	REPS ☐	REPS ☐
	WEIGHT				
		REPS ☐	REPS ☐	REPS ☐	REPS ☐
	WEIGHT				

EXERCISE	SETS	REPS AND DONE!				
		REPS ☐	REPS ☐	REPS ☐	REPS ☐	REPS ☐
	WEIGHT					
		REPS ☐	REPS ☐	REPS ☐	REPS ☐	REPS ☐
	WEIGHT					
		REPS ☐	REPS ☐	REPS ☐	REPS ☐	REPS ☐
	WEIGHT					
		REPS ☐	REPS ☐	REPS ☐	REPS ☐	REPS ☐
	WEIGHT					
		REPS ☐	REPS ☐	REPS ☐	REPS ☐	REPS ☐
	WEIGHT					
		REPS ☐	REPS ☐	REPS ☐	REPS ☐	REPS ☐
	WEIGHT					
		REPS ☐	REPS ☐	REPS ☐	REPS ☐	REPS ☐
	WEIGHT					
		REPS ☐	REPS ☐	REPS ☐	REPS ☐	REPS ☐
	WEIGHT					
		REPS ☐	REPS ☐	REPS ☐	REPS ☐	REPS ☐
	WEIGHT					
		REPS ☐	REPS ☐	REPS ☐	REPS ☐	REPS ☐
	WEIGHT					
		REPS ☐	REPS ☐	REPS ☐	REPS ☐	REPS ☐
	WEIGHT					

		REPS ☐	REPS ☐	REPS ☐	REPS ☐
WEIGHT 〔〕–〔〕→					
		REPS ☐	REPS ☐	REPS ☐	REPS ☐
WEIGHT 〔〕–〔〕→					
		REPS ☐	REPS ☐	REPS ☐	REPS ☐
WEIGHT 〔〕–〔〕→					
		REPS ☐	REPS ☐	REPS ☐	REPS ☐
WEIGHT 〔〕–〔〕→					
		REPS ☐	REPS ☐	REPS ☐	REPS ☐
WEIGHT 〔〕–〔〕→					
		REPS ☐	REPS ☐	REPS ☐	REPS ☐
WEIGHT 〔〕–〔〕→					
		REPS ☐	REPS ☐	REPS ☐	REPS ☐
WEIGHT 〔〕–〔〕→					
		REPS ☐	REPS ☐	REPS ☐	REPS ☐
WEIGHT 〔〕–〔〕→					
		REPS ☐	REPS ☐	REPS ☐	REPS ☐
WEIGHT 〔〕–〔〕→					
		REPS ☐	REPS ☐	REPS ☐	REPS ☐
WEIGHT 〔〕–〔〕→					

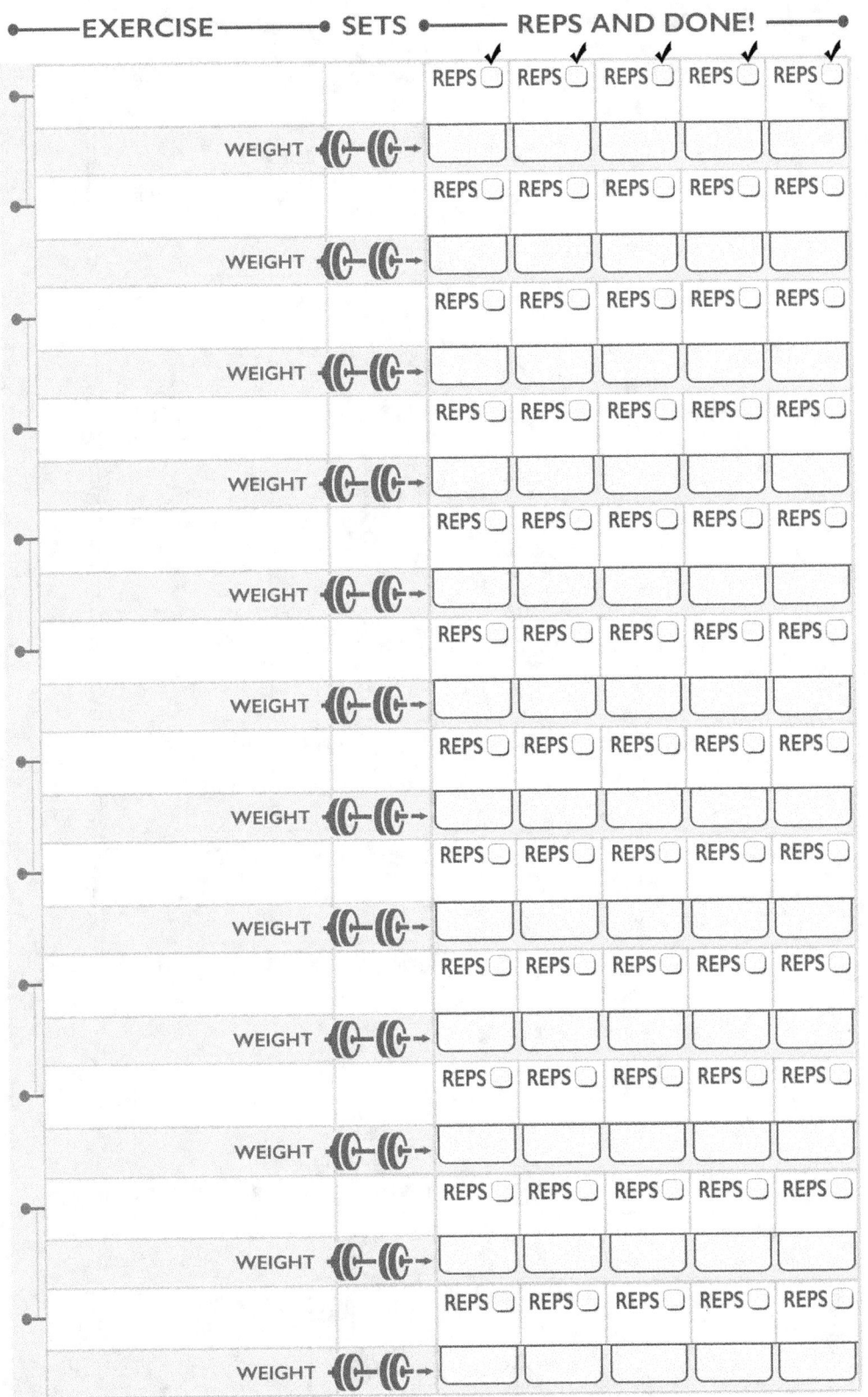

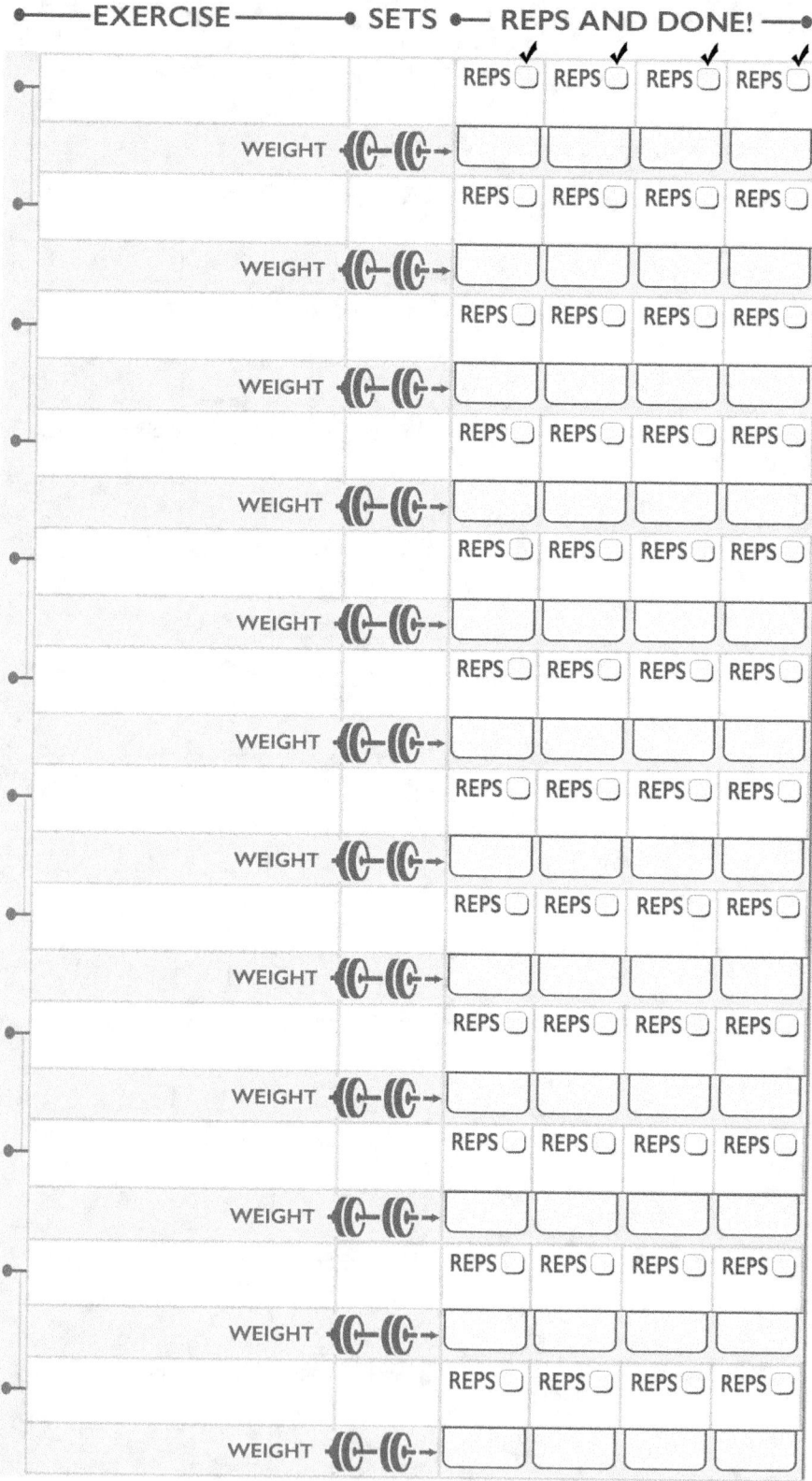

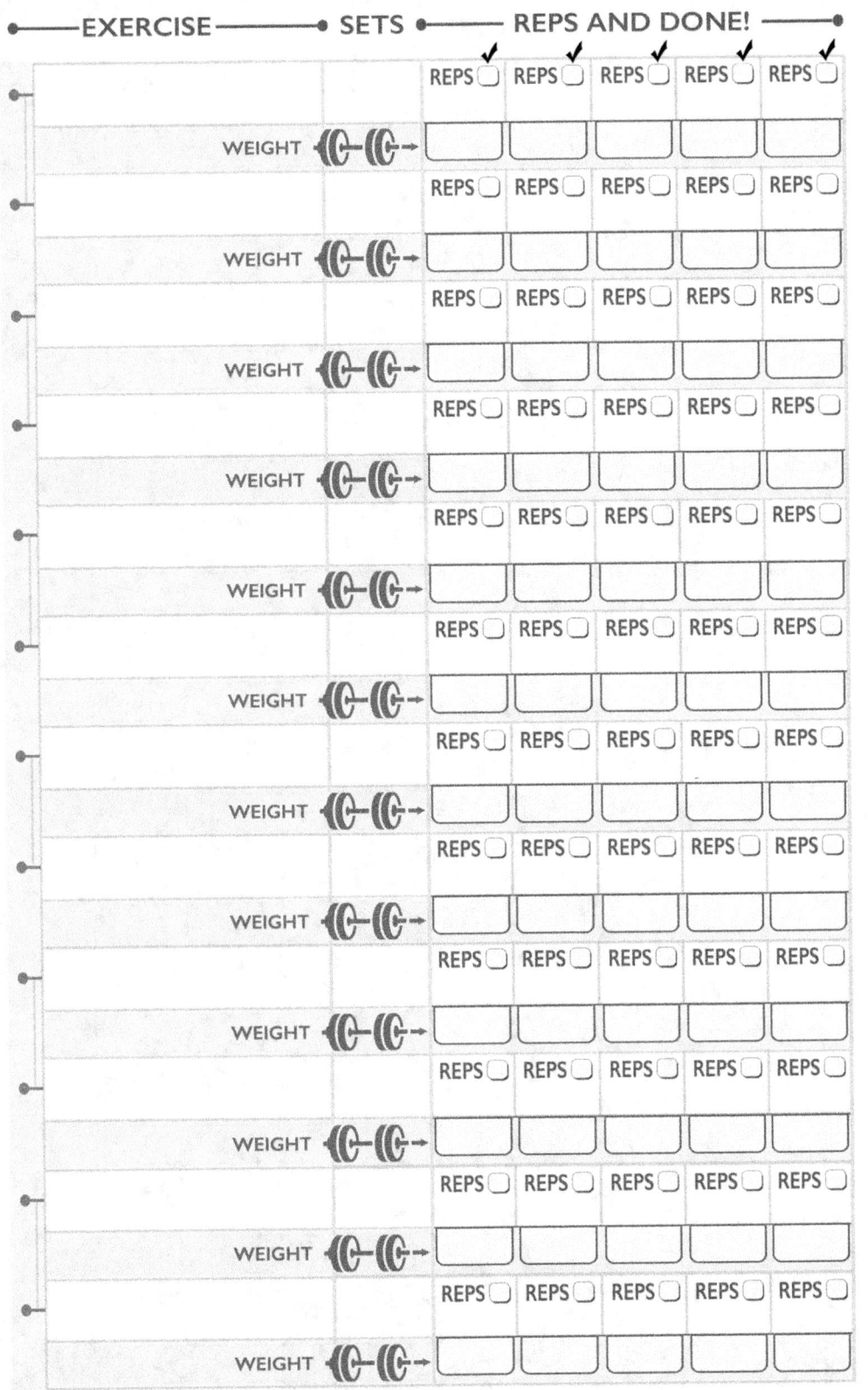

EXERCISE ——— SETS ——— REPS AND DONE! ———

EXERCISE	SETS	REPS ✓	REPS ✓	REPS ✓	REPS ✓
	WEIGHT				
		REPS ☐	REPS ☐	REPS ☐	REPS ☐
	WEIGHT				
		REPS ☐	REPS ☐	REPS ☐	REPS ☐
	WEIGHT				
		REPS ☐	REPS ☐	REPS ☐	REPS ☐
	WEIGHT				
		REPS ☐	REPS ☐	REPS ☐	REPS ☐
	WEIGHT				
		REPS ☐	REPS ☐	REPS ☐	REPS ☐
	WEIGHT				
		REPS ☐	REPS ☐	REPS ☐	REPS ☐
	WEIGHT				
		REPS ☐	REPS ☐	REPS ☐	REPS ☐
	WEIGHT				
		REPS ☐	REPS ☐	REPS ☐	REPS ☐
	WEIGHT				
		REPS ☐	REPS ☐	REPS ☐	REPS ☐
	WEIGHT				
		REPS ☐	REPS ☐	REPS ☐	REPS ☐
	WEIGHT				

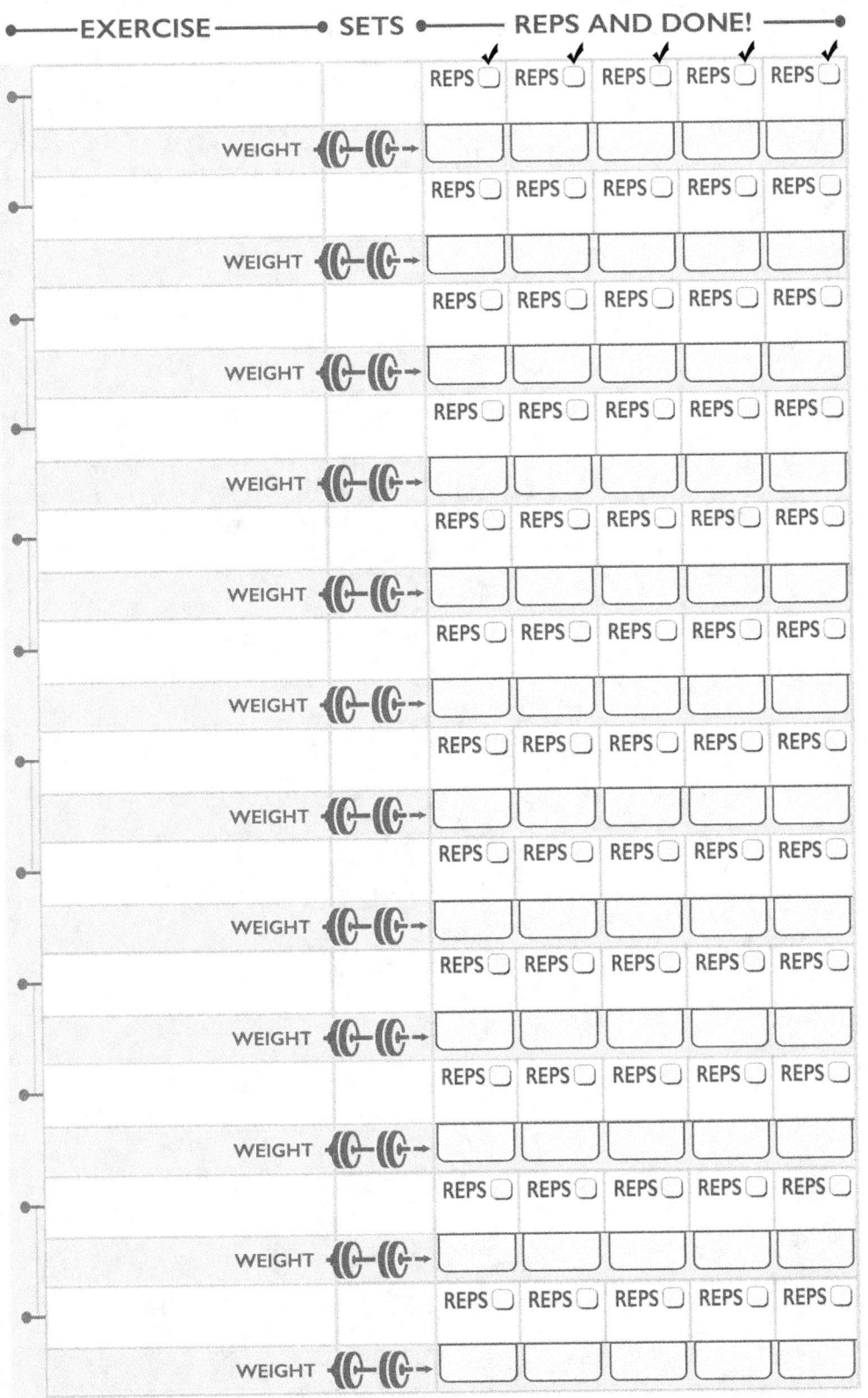

EXERCISE	SETS	REPS ☑	REPS ☑	REPS ☑	REPS ☑
	WEIGHT				
		REPS ☐	REPS ☐	REPS ☐	REPS ☐
	WEIGHT				
		REPS ☐	REPS ☐	REPS ☐	REPS ☐
	WEIGHT				
		REPS ☐	REPS ☐	REPS ☐	REPS ☐
	WEIGHT				
		REPS ☐	REPS ☐	REPS ☐	REPS ☐
	WEIGHT				
		REPS ☐	REPS ☐	REPS ☐	REPS ☐
	WEIGHT				
		REPS ☐	REPS ☐	REPS ☐	REPS ☐
	WEIGHT				
		REPS ☐	REPS ☐	REPS ☐	REPS ☐
	WEIGHT				
		REPS ☐	REPS ☐	REPS ☐	REPS ☐
	WEIGHT				
		REPS ☐	REPS ☐	REPS ☐	REPS ☐
	WEIGHT				
		REPS ☐	REPS ☐	REPS ☐	REPS ☐
	WEIGHT				

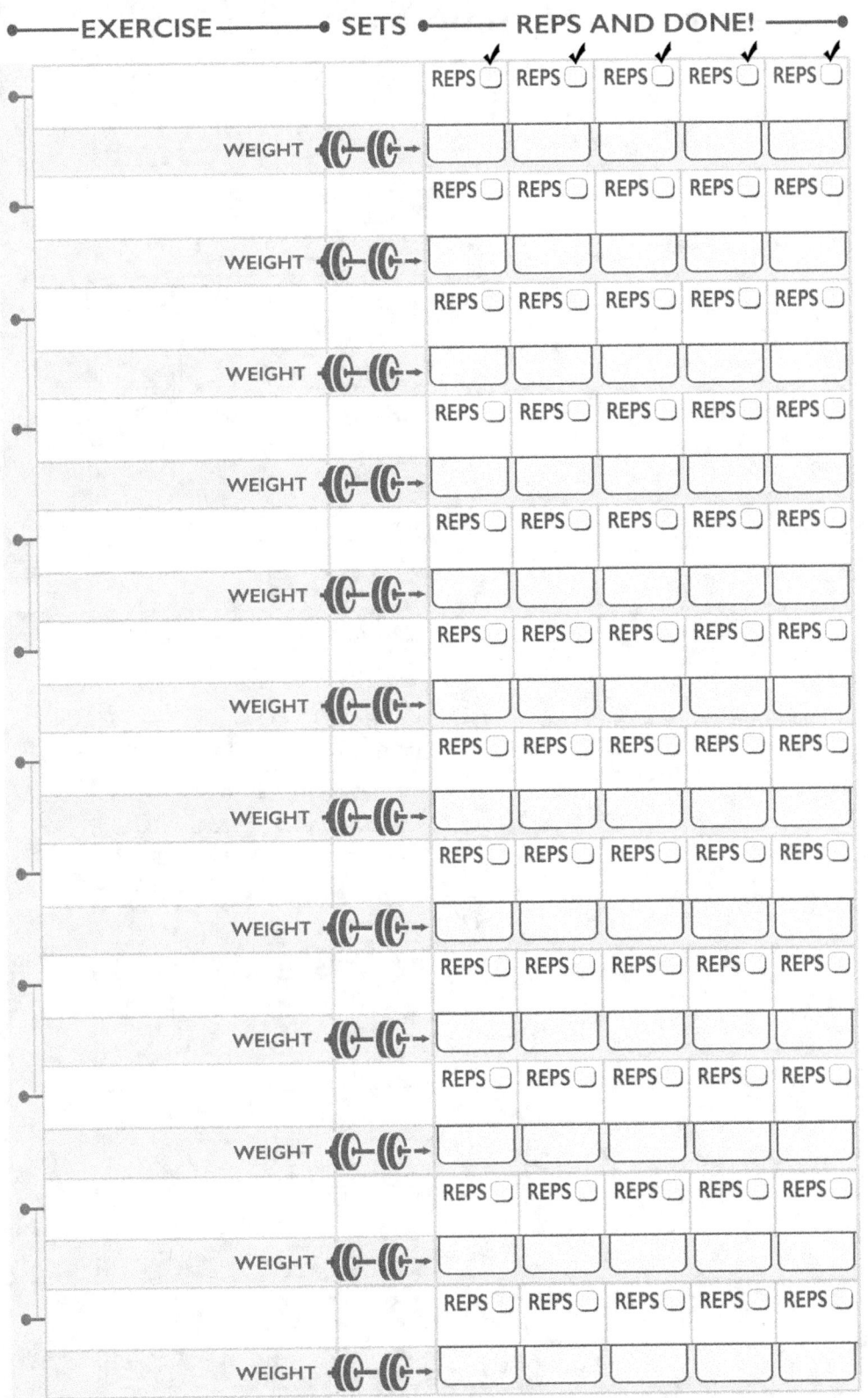

EXERCISE	SETS	REPS ✓	REPS ✓	REPS ✓	REPS ✓
	WEIGHT				
		REPS	REPS	REPS	REPS
	WEIGHT				
		REPS	REPS	REPS	REPS
	WEIGHT				
		REPS	REPS	REPS	REPS
	WEIGHT				
		REPS	REPS	REPS	REPS
	WEIGHT				
		REPS	REPS	REPS	REPS
	WEIGHT				
		REPS	REPS	REPS	REPS
	WEIGHT				
		REPS	REPS	REPS	REPS
	WEIGHT				
		REPS	REPS	REPS	REPS
	WEIGHT				
		REPS	REPS	REPS	REPS
	WEIGHT				

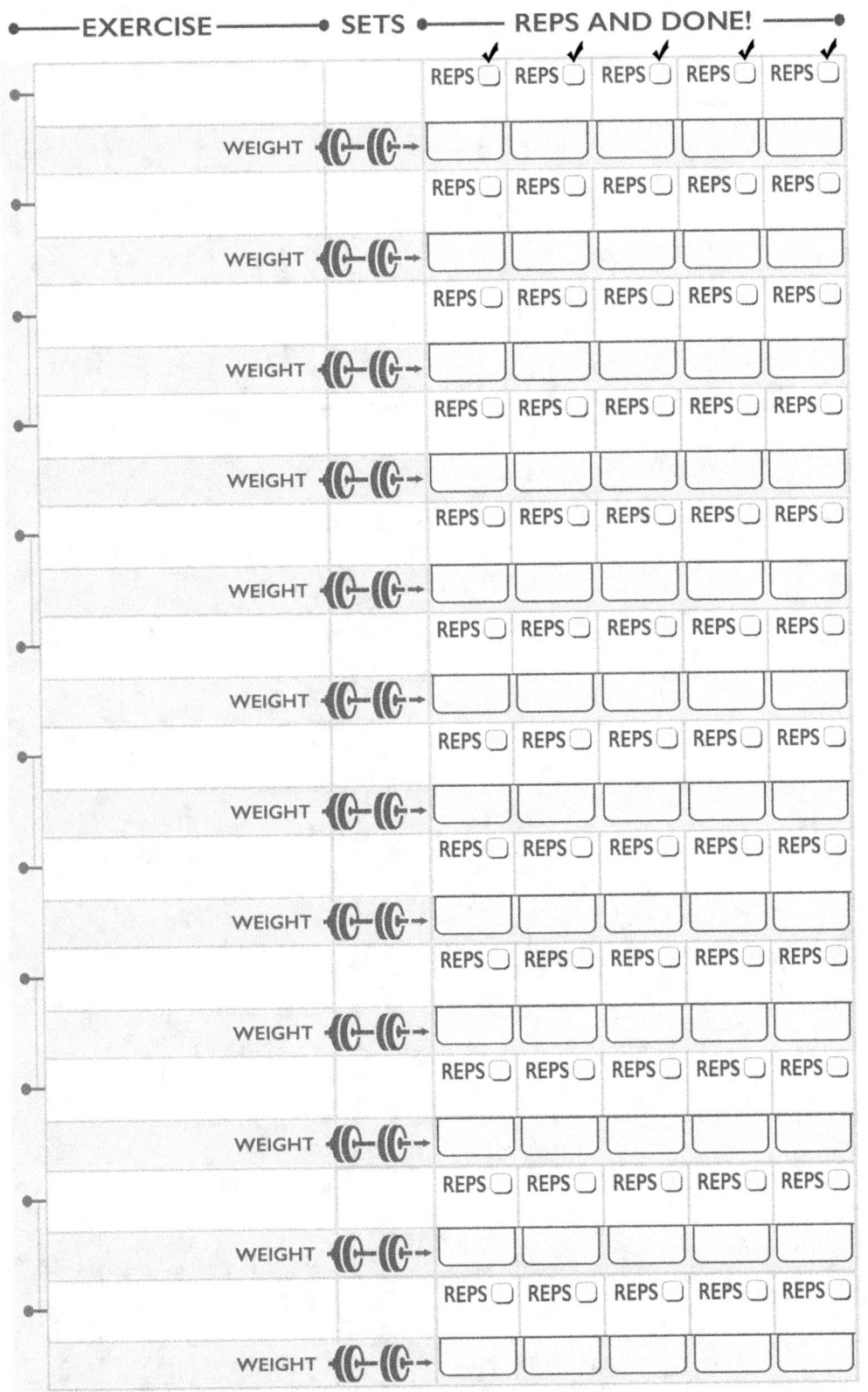

EXERCISE — SETS — REPS AND DONE! —

		REPS ☐	REPS ☐	REPS ☐	REPS ☐	REPS ☐
	WEIGHT					
		REPS ☐	REPS ☐	REPS ☐	REPS ☐	REPS ☐
	WEIGHT					
		REPS ☐	REPS ☐	REPS ☐	REPS ☐	REPS ☐
	WEIGHT					
		REPS ☐	REPS ☐	REPS ☐	REPS ☐	REPS ☐
	WEIGHT					
		REPS ☐	REPS ☐	REPS ☐	REPS ☐	REPS ☐
	WEIGHT					
		REPS ☐	REPS ☐	REPS ☐	REPS ☐	REPS ☐
	WEIGHT					
		REPS ☐	REPS ☐	REPS ☐	REPS ☐	REPS ☐
	WEIGHT					
		REPS ☐	REPS ☐	REPS ☐	REPS ☐	REPS ☐
	WEIGHT					
		REPS ☐	REPS ☐	REPS ☐	REPS ☐	REPS ☐
	WEIGHT					
		REPS ☐	REPS ☐	REPS ☐	REPS ☐	REPS ☐
	WEIGHT					

EXERCISE	SETS	REPS AND DONE!			
		REPS ☐	REPS ☐	REPS ☐	REPS ☐
	WEIGHT ◀█─█▶				
		REPS ☐	REPS ☐	REPS ☐	REPS ☐
	WEIGHT ◀█─█▶				
		REPS ☐	REPS ☐	REPS ☐	REPS ☐
	WEIGHT ◀█─█▶				
		REPS ☐	REPS ☐	REPS ☐	REPS ☐
	WEIGHT ◀█─█▶				
		REPS ☐	REPS ☐	REPS ☐	REPS ☐
	WEIGHT ◀█─█▶				
		REPS ☐	REPS ☐	REPS ☐	REPS ☐
	WEIGHT ◀█─█▶				
		REPS ☐	REPS ☐	REPS ☐	REPS ☐
	WEIGHT ◀█─█▶				
		REPS ☐	REPS ☐	REPS ☐	REPS ☐
	WEIGHT ◀█─█▶				
		REPS ☐	REPS ☐	REPS ☐	REPS ☐
	WEIGHT ◀█─█▶				
		REPS ☐	REPS ☐	REPS ☐	REPS ☐
	WEIGHT ◀█─█▶				

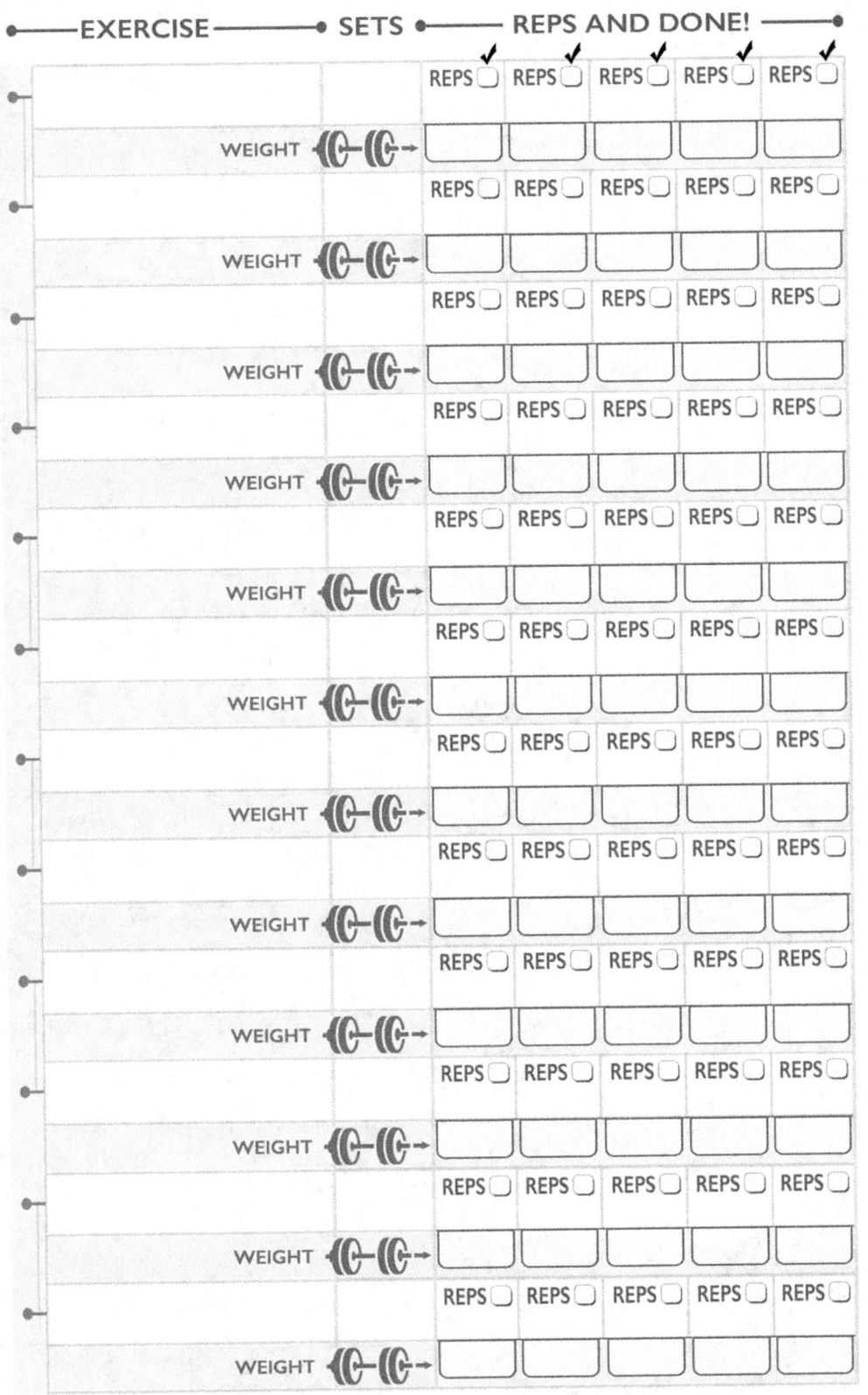

		REPS ☐	REPS ☐	REPS ☐	REPS ☐
WEIGHT ◖◖-◖◖→					
		REPS ☐	REPS ☐	REPS ☐	REPS ☐
WEIGHT ◖◖-◖◖→					
		REPS ☐	REPS ☐	REPS ☐	REPS ☐
WEIGHT ◖◖-◖◖→					
		REPS ☐	REPS ☐	REPS ☐	REPS ☐
WEIGHT ◖◖-◖◖→					
		REPS ☐	REPS ☐	REPS ☐	REPS ☐
WEIGHT ◖◖-◖◖→					
		REPS ☐	REPS ☐	REPS ☐	REPS ☐
WEIGHT ◖◖-◖◖→					
		REPS ☐	REPS ☐	REPS ☐	REPS ☐
WEIGHT ◖◖-◖◖→					
		REPS ☐	REPS ☐	REPS ☐	REPS ☐
WEIGHT ◖◖-◖◖→					
		REPS ☐	REPS ☐	REPS ☐	REPS ☐
WEIGHT ◖◖-◖◖→					
		REPS ☐	REPS ☐	REPS ☐	REPS ☐
WEIGHT ◖◖-◖◖→					

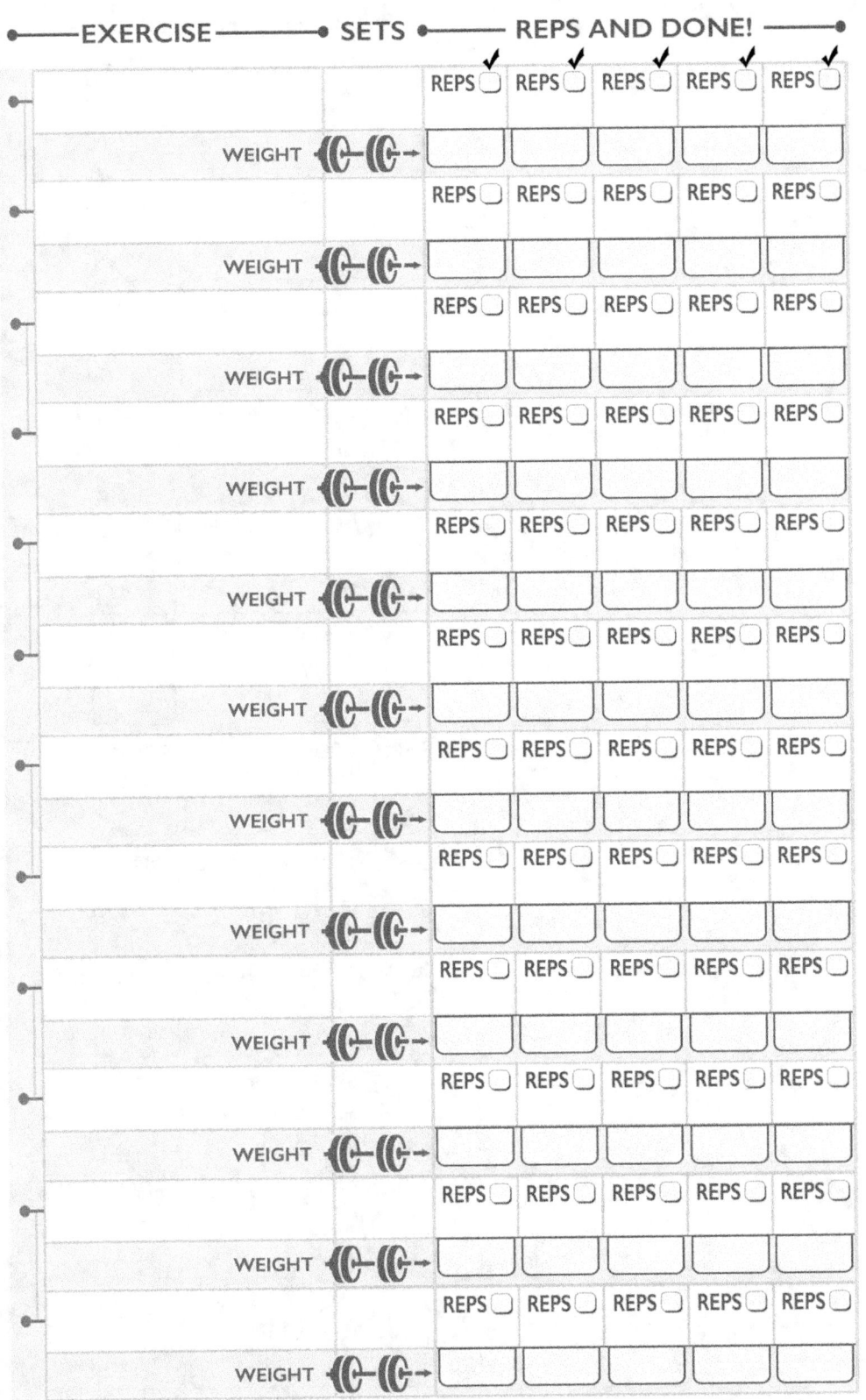

EXERCISE	SETS	REPS ✓	REPS ✓	REPS ✓	REPS ✓
	WEIGHT				
		REPS	REPS	REPS	REPS
	WEIGHT				
		REPS	REPS	REPS	REPS
	WEIGHT				
		REPS	REPS	REPS	REPS
	WEIGHT				
		REPS	REPS	REPS	REPS
	WEIGHT				
		REPS	REPS	REPS	REPS
	WEIGHT				
		REPS	REPS	REPS	REPS
	WEIGHT				
		REPS	REPS	REPS	REPS
	WEIGHT				
		REPS	REPS	REPS	REPS
	WEIGHT				
		REPS	REPS	REPS	REPS
	WEIGHT				
		REPS	REPS	REPS	REPS
	WEIGHT				

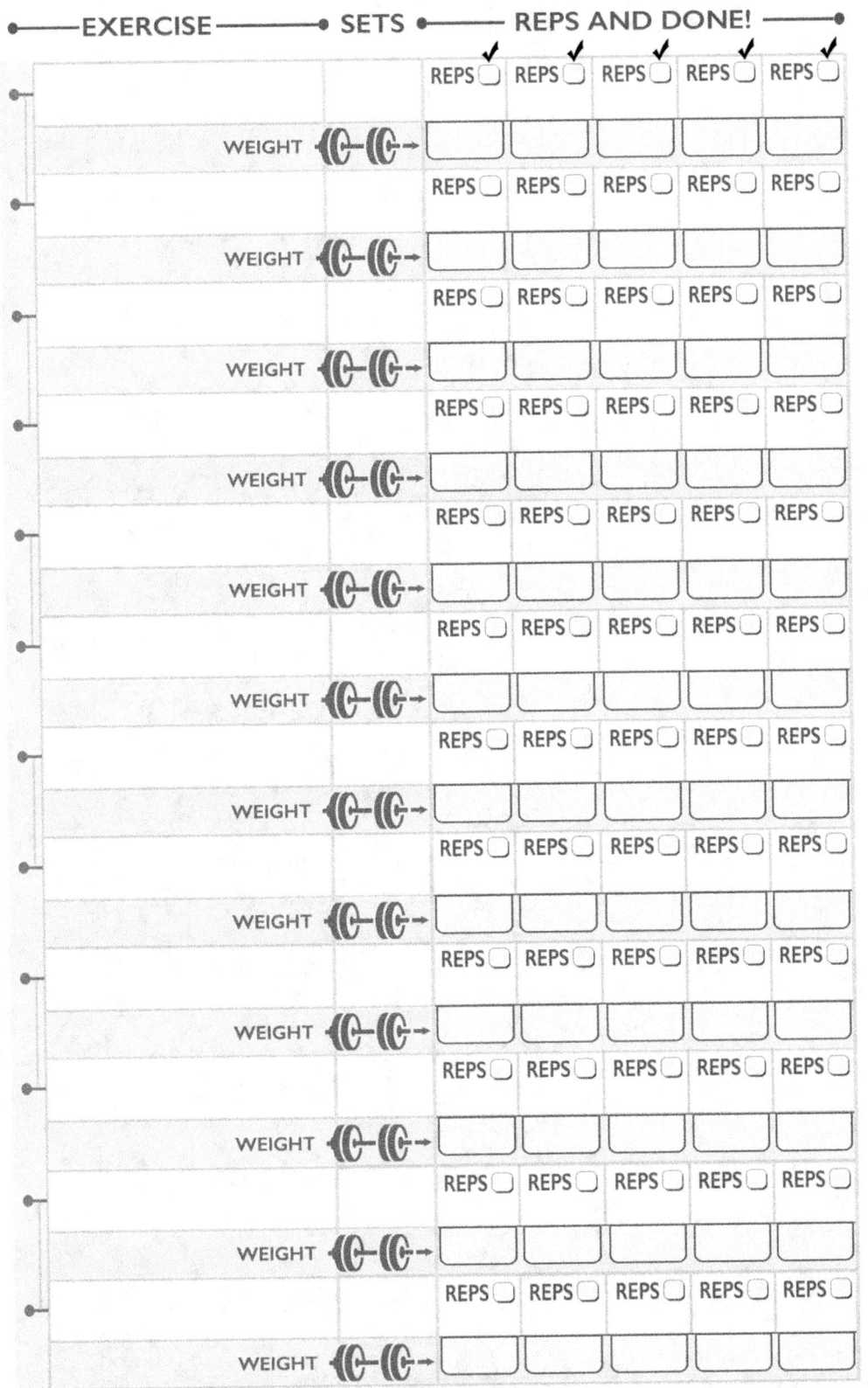

EXERCISE	SETS	REPS AND DONE!			
		REPS ☐	REPS ☐	REPS ☐	REPS ☐
	WEIGHT 〈€–€〉→				
		REPS ☐	REPS ☐	REPS ☐	REPS ☐
	WEIGHT 〈€–€〉→				
		REPS ☐	REPS ☐	REPS ☐	REPS ☐
	WEIGHT 〈€–€〉→				
		REPS ☐	REPS ☐	REPS ☐	REPS ☐
	WEIGHT 〈€–€〉→				
		REPS ☐	REPS ☐	REPS ☐	REPS ☐
	WEIGHT 〈€–€〉→				
		REPS ☐	REPS ☐	REPS ☐	REPS ☐
	WEIGHT 〈€–€〉→				
		REPS ☐	REPS ☐	REPS ☐	REPS ☐
	WEIGHT 〈€–€〉→				
		REPS ☐	REPS ☐	REPS ☐	REPS ☐
	WEIGHT 〈€–€〉→				
		REPS ☐	REPS ☐	REPS ☐	REPS ☐
	WEIGHT 〈€–€〉→				
		REPS ☐	REPS ☐	REPS ☐	REPS ☐
	WEIGHT 〈€–€〉→				
		REPS ☐	REPS ☐	REPS ☐	REPS ☐
	WEIGHT 〈€–€〉→				

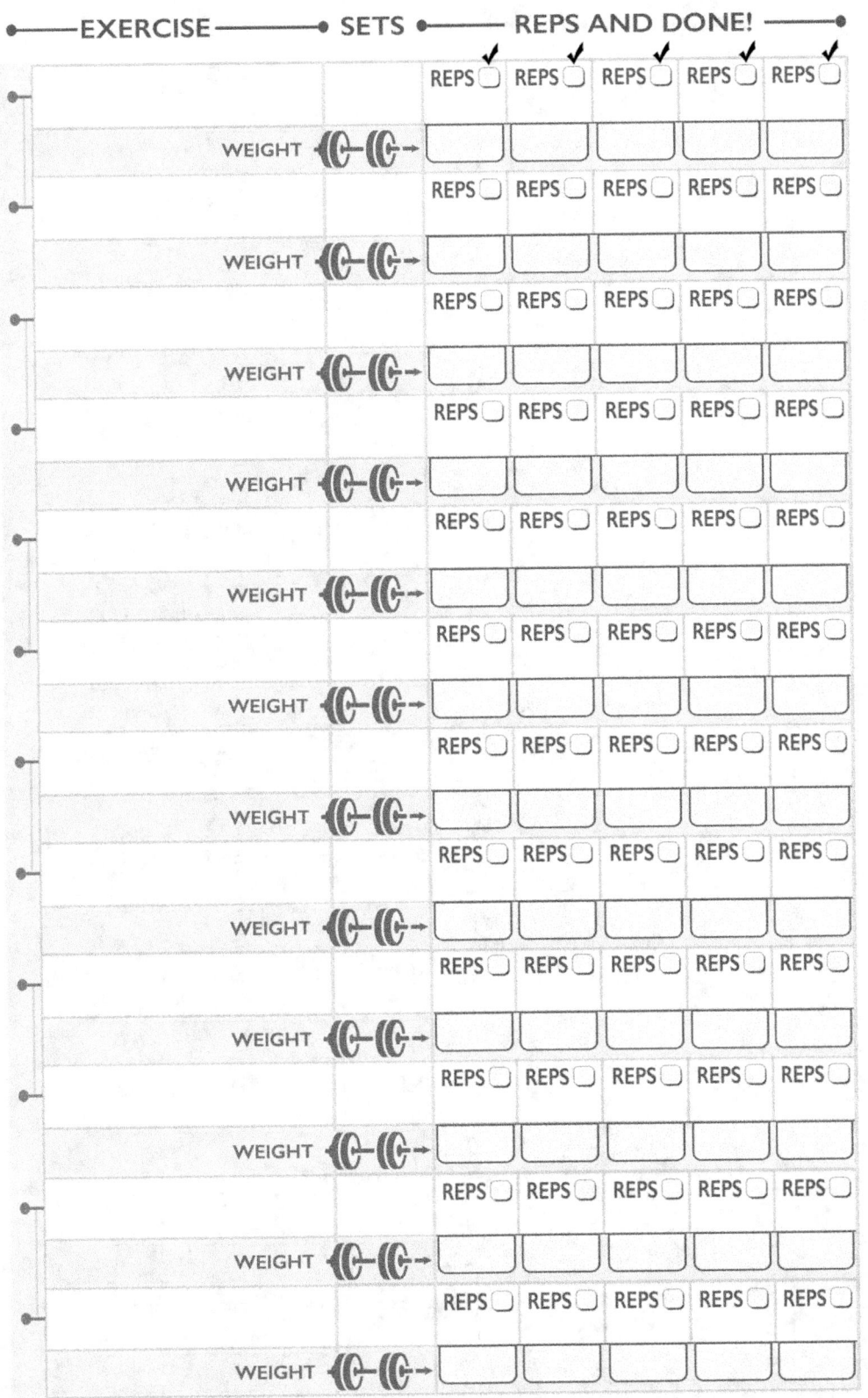

EXERCISE	SETS	REPS ✓	REPS ✓	REPS ✓	REPS ✓
	WEIGHT				
		REPS	REPS	REPS	REPS
	WEIGHT				
		REPS	REPS	REPS	REPS
	WEIGHT				
		REPS	REPS	REPS	REPS
	WEIGHT				
		REPS	REPS	REPS	REPS
	WEIGHT				
		REPS	REPS	REPS	REPS
	WEIGHT				
		REPS	REPS	REPS	REPS
	WEIGHT				
		REPS	REPS	REPS	REPS
	WEIGHT				
		REPS	REPS	REPS	REPS
	WEIGHT				
		REPS	REPS	REPS	REPS
	WEIGHT				

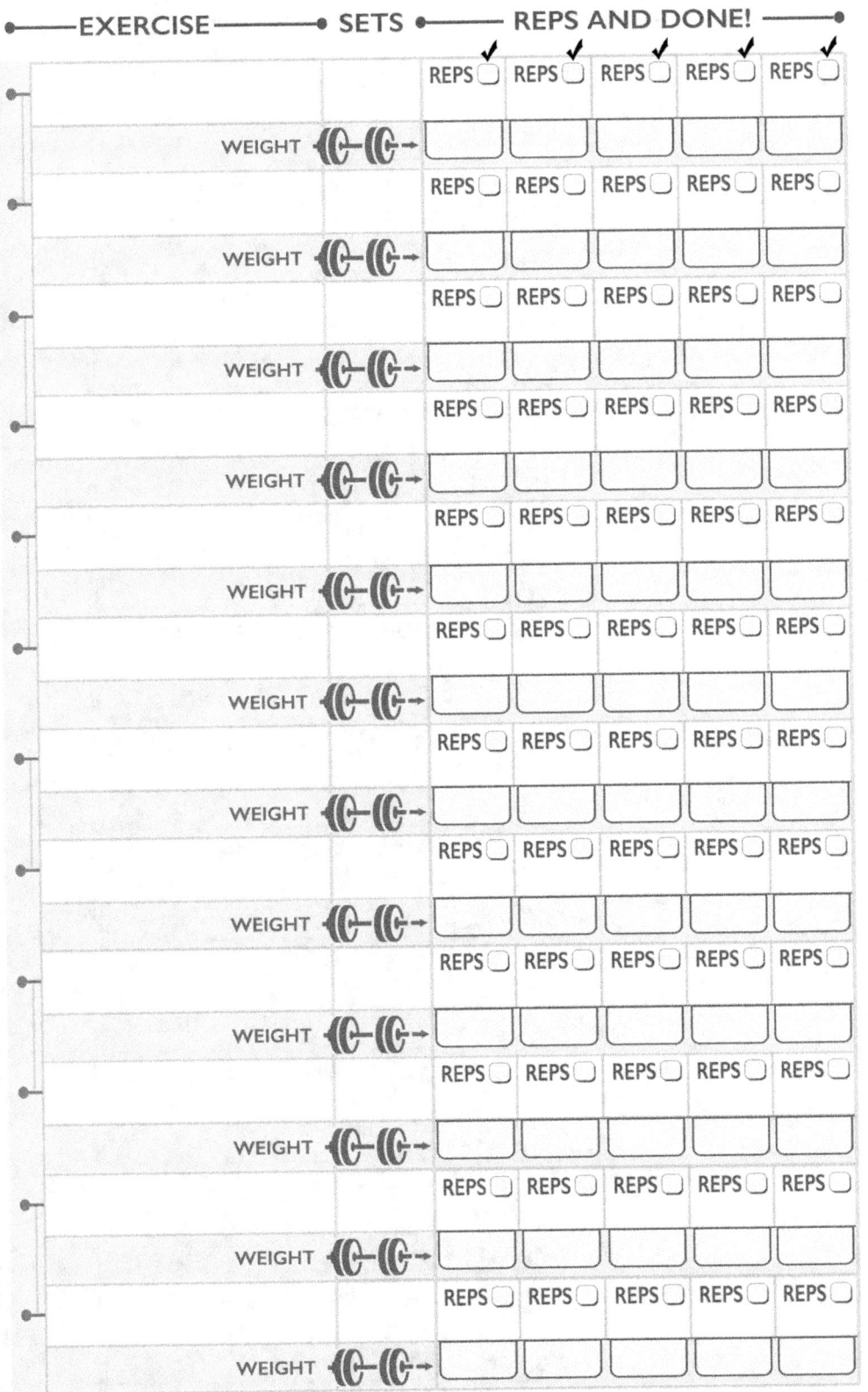

EXERCISE	SETS	REPS ✓	REPS ✓	REPS ✓	REPS ✓
	WEIGHT ⬦–⬦→				
		REPS ◯	REPS ◯	REPS ◯	REPS ◯
	WEIGHT ⬦–⬦→				
		REPS ◯	REPS ◯	REPS ◯	REPS ◯
	WEIGHT ⬦–⬦→				
		REPS ◯	REPS ◯	REPS ◯	REPS ◯
	WEIGHT ⬦–⬦→				
		REPS ◯	REPS ◯	REPS ◯	REPS ◯
	WEIGHT ⬦–⬦→				
		REPS ◯	REPS ◯	REPS ◯	REPS ◯
	WEIGHT ⬦–⬦→				
		REPS ◯	REPS ◯	REPS ◯	REPS ◯
	WEIGHT ⬦–⬦→				
		REPS ◯	REPS ◯	REPS ◯	REPS ◯
	WEIGHT ⬦–⬦→				
		REPS ◯	REPS ◯	REPS ◯	REPS ◯
	WEIGHT ⬦–⬦→				
		REPS ◯	REPS ◯	REPS ◯	REPS ◯
	WEIGHT ⬦–⬦→				
		REPS ◯	REPS ◯	REPS ◯	REPS ◯
	WEIGHT ⬦–⬦→				

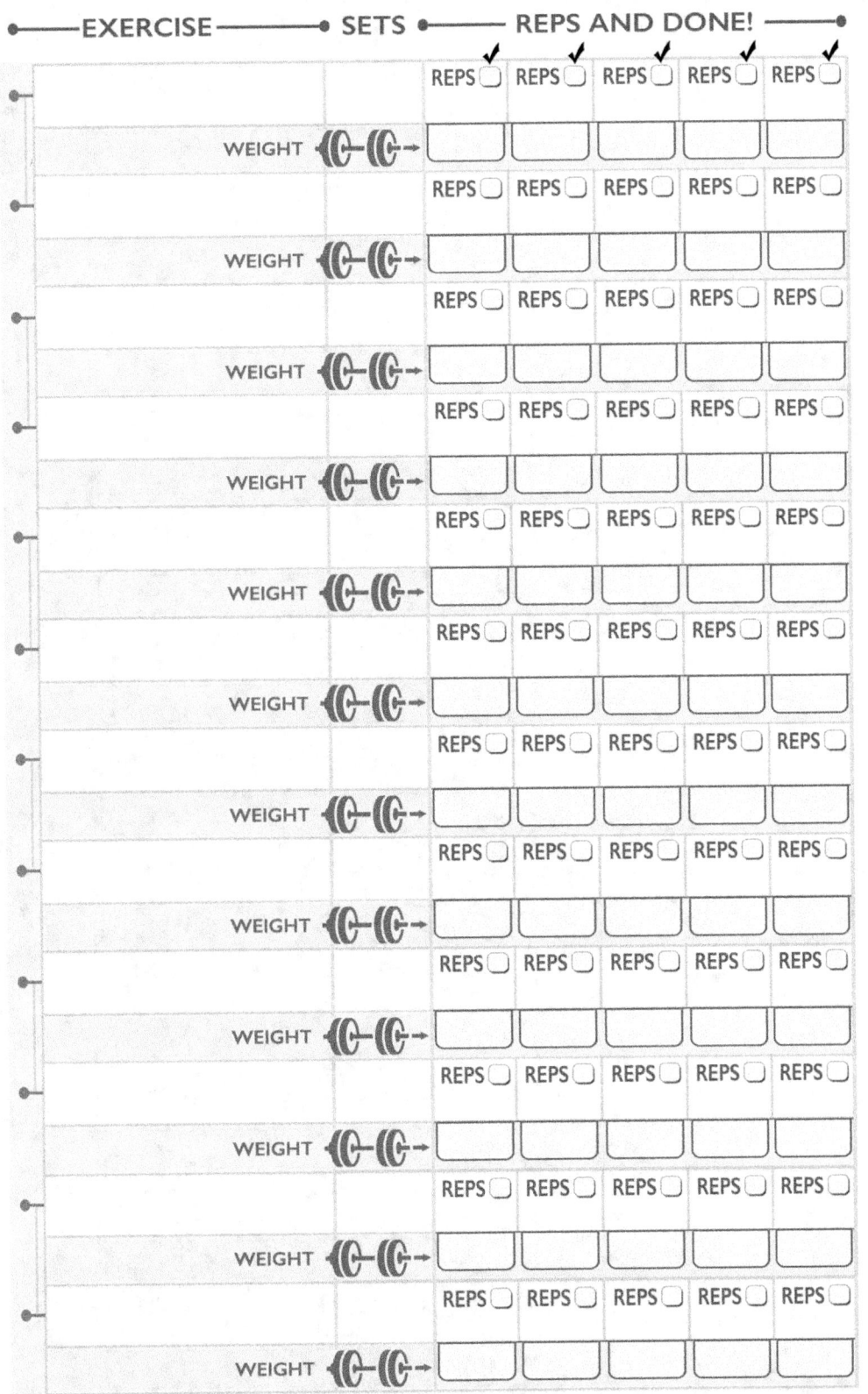

EXERCISE	SETS	REPS AND DONE!			
		REPS ☐	REPS ☐	REPS ☐	REPS ☐
	WEIGHT				
		REPS ☐	REPS ☐	REPS ☐	REPS ☐
	WEIGHT				
		REPS ☐	REPS ☐	REPS ☐	REPS ☐
	WEIGHT				
		REPS ☐	REPS ☐	REPS ☐	REPS ☐
	WEIGHT				
		REPS ☐	REPS ☐	REPS ☐	REPS ☐
	WEIGHT				
		REPS ☐	REPS ☐	REPS ☐	REPS ☐
	WEIGHT				
		REPS ☐	REPS ☐	REPS ☐	REPS ☐
	WEIGHT				
		REPS ☐	REPS ☐	REPS ☐	REPS ☐
	WEIGHT				
		REPS ☐	REPS ☐	REPS ☐	REPS ☐
	WEIGHT				
		REPS ☐	REPS ☐	REPS ☐	REPS ☐
	WEIGHT				
		REPS ☐	REPS ☐	REPS ☐	REPS ☐
	WEIGHT				

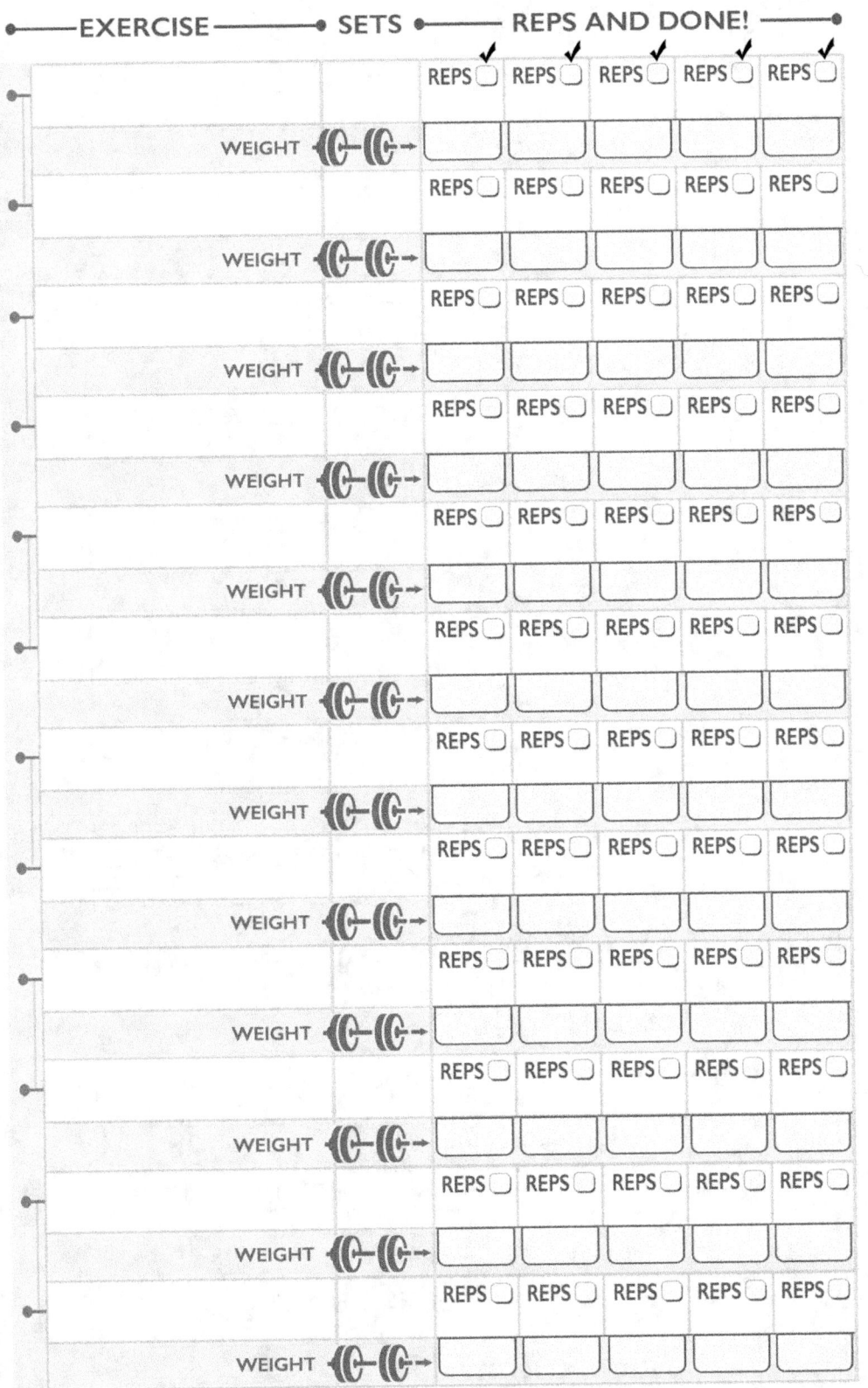

		REPS ☐	REPS ☐	REPS ☐	REPS ☐
WEIGHT					
		REPS ☐	REPS ☐	REPS ☐	REPS ☐
WEIGHT					
		REPS ☐	REPS ☐	REPS ☐	REPS ☐
WEIGHT					
		REPS ☐	REPS ☐	REPS ☐	REPS ☐
WEIGHT					
		REPS ☐	REPS ☐	REPS ☐	REPS ☐
WEIGHT					
		REPS ☐	REPS ☐	REPS ☐	REPS ☐
WEIGHT					
		REPS ☐	REPS ☐	REPS ☐	REPS ☐
WEIGHT					
		REPS ☐	REPS ☐	REPS ☐	REPS ☐
WEIGHT					
		REPS ☐	REPS ☐	REPS ☐	REPS ☐
WEIGHT					
		REPS ☐	REPS ☐	REPS ☐	REPS ☐
WEIGHT					

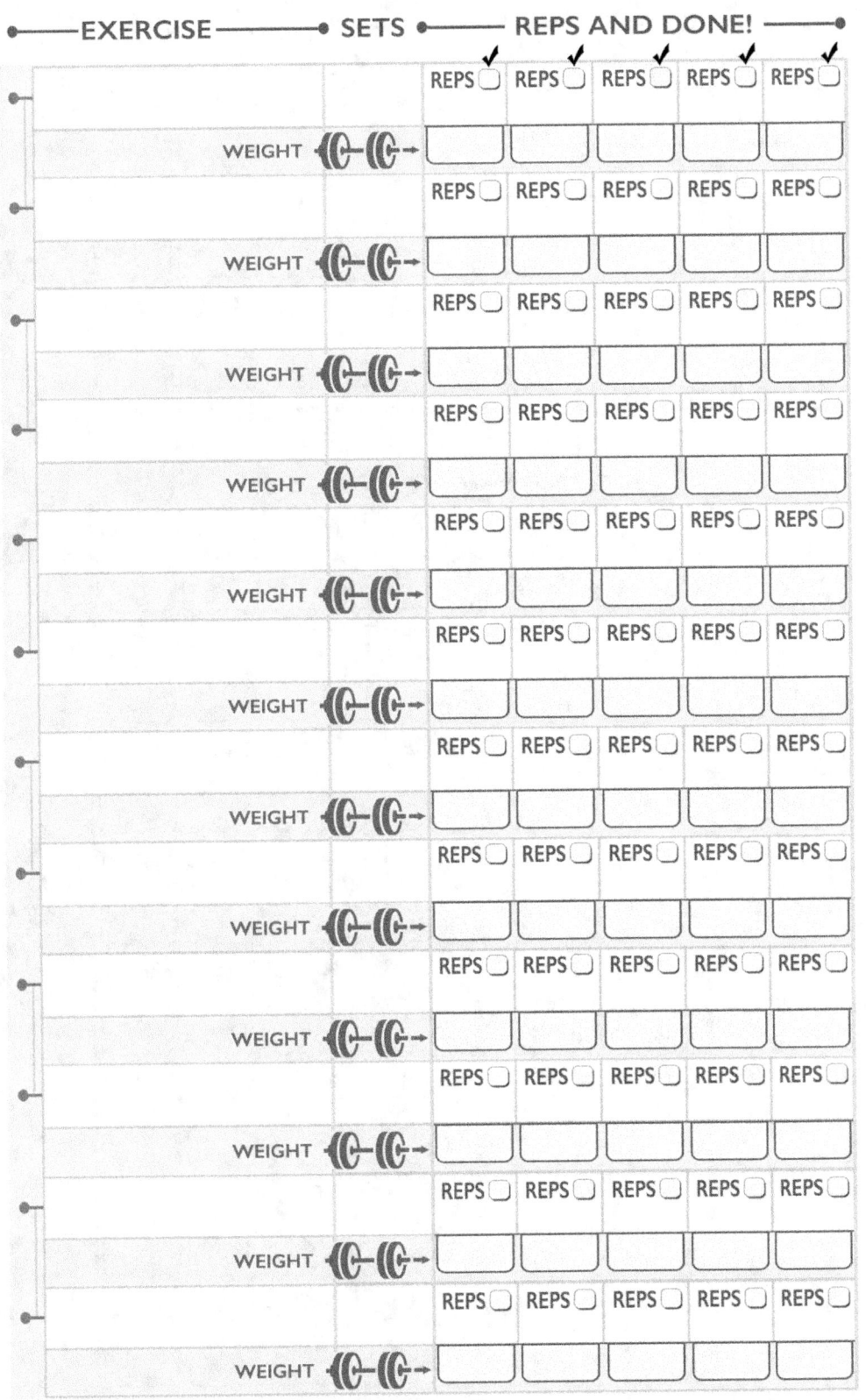

EXERCISE	SETS	REPS ✓	REPS ✓	REPS ✓	REPS ✓
	WEIGHT				
		REPS	REPS	REPS	REPS
	WEIGHT				
		REPS	REPS	REPS	REPS
	WEIGHT				
		REPS	REPS	REPS	REPS
	WEIGHT				
		REPS	REPS	REPS	REPS
	WEIGHT				
		REPS	REPS	REPS	REPS
	WEIGHT				
		REPS	REPS	REPS	REPS
	WEIGHT				
		REPS	REPS	REPS	REPS
	WEIGHT				
		REPS	REPS	REPS	REPS
	WEIGHT				
		REPS	REPS	REPS	REPS
	WEIGHT				

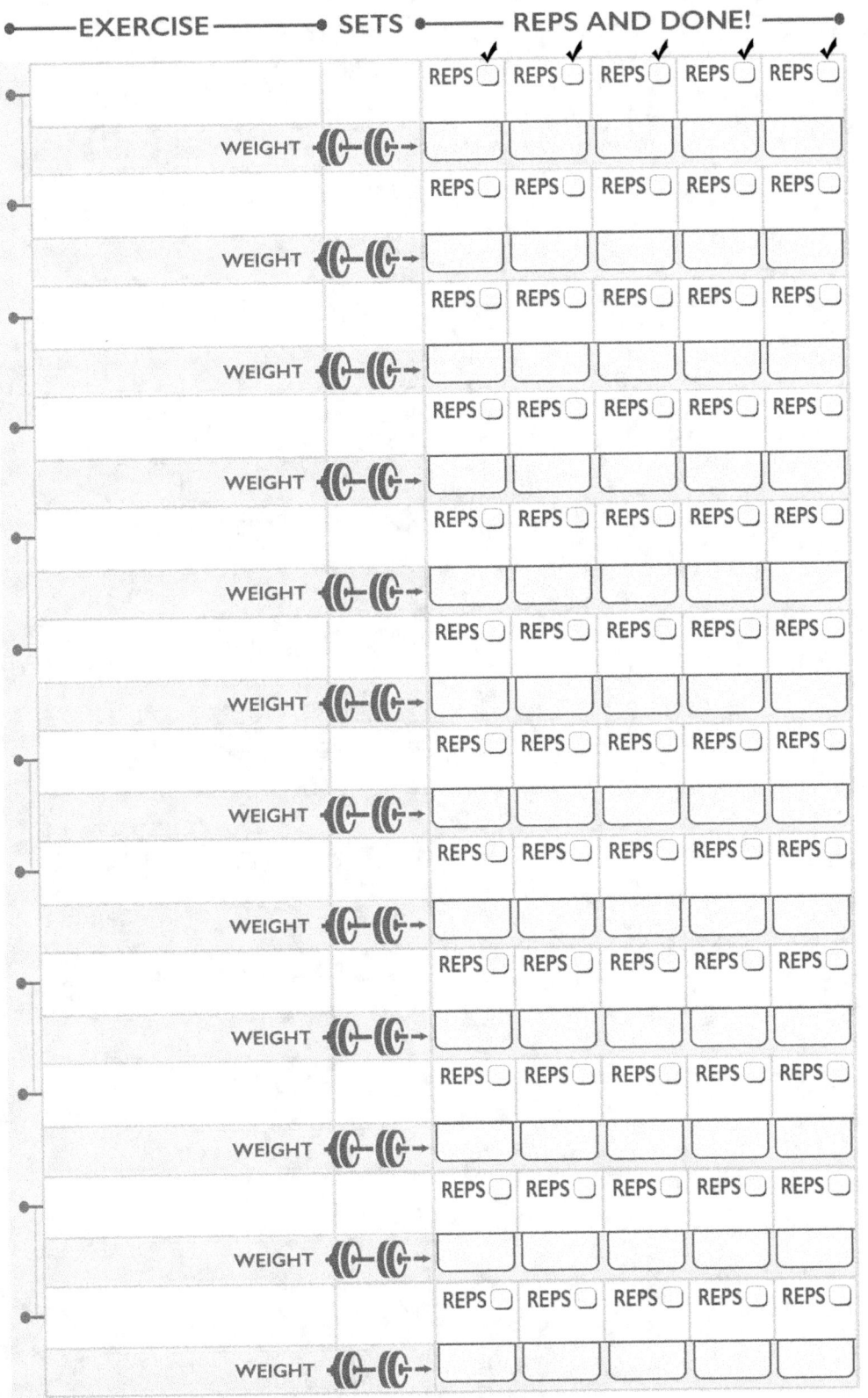

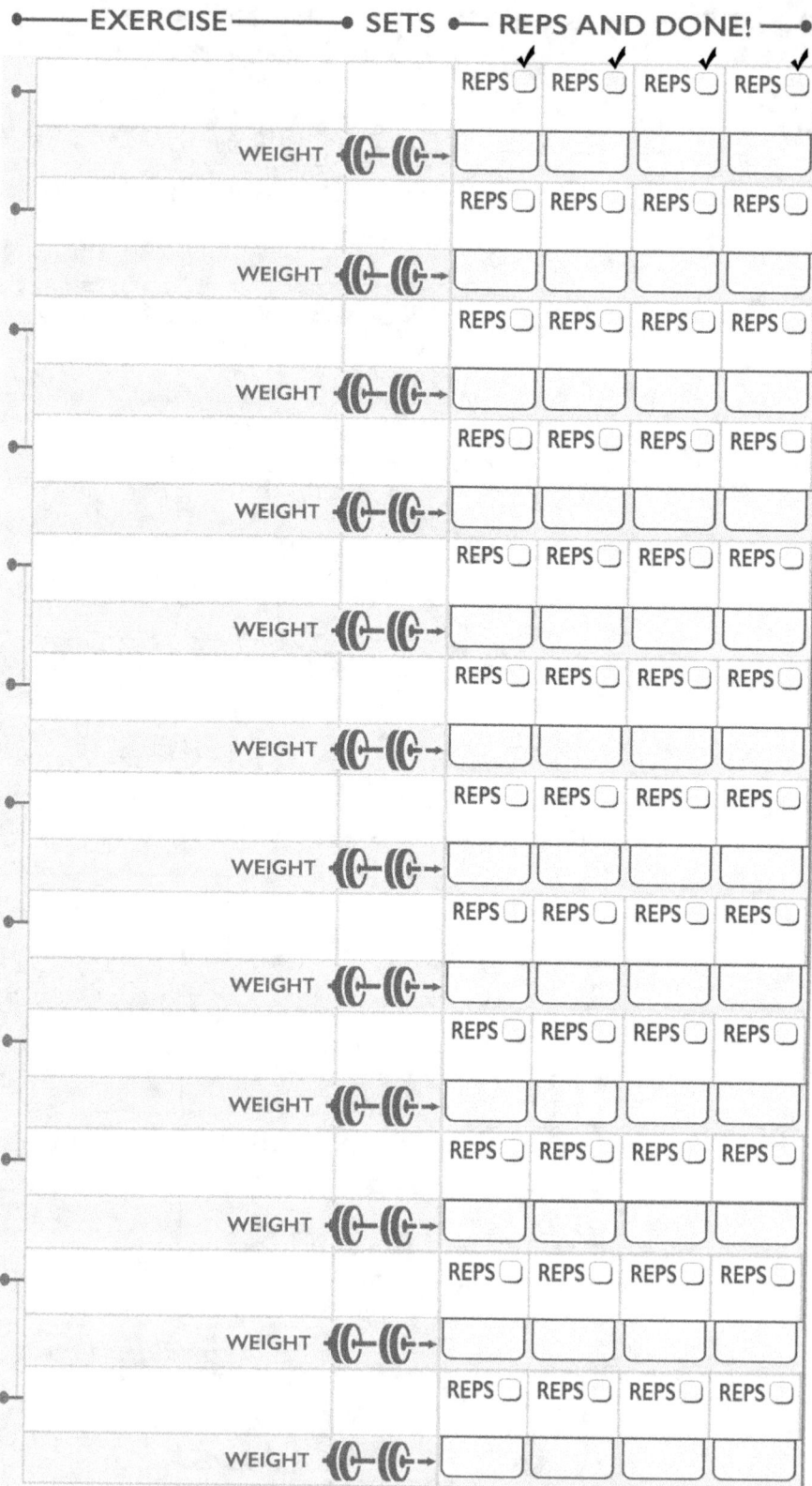

		REPS ☐	REPS ☐	REPS ☐	REPS ☐
	WEIGHT				
		REPS ☐	REPS ☐	REPS ☐	REPS ☐
	WEIGHT				
		REPS ☐	REPS ☐	REPS ☐	REPS ☐
	WEIGHT				
		REPS ☐	REPS ☐	REPS ☐	REPS ☐
	WEIGHT				
		REPS ☐	REPS ☐	REPS ☐	REPS ☐
	WEIGHT				
		REPS ☐	REPS ☐	REPS ☐	REPS ☐
	WEIGHT				
		REPS ☐	REPS ☐	REPS ☐	REPS ☐
	WEIGHT				
		REPS ☐	REPS ☐	REPS ☐	REPS ☐
	WEIGHT				
		REPS ☐	REPS ☐	REPS ☐	REPS ☐
	WEIGHT				
		REPS ☐	REPS ☐	REPS ☐	REPS ☐
	WEIGHT				

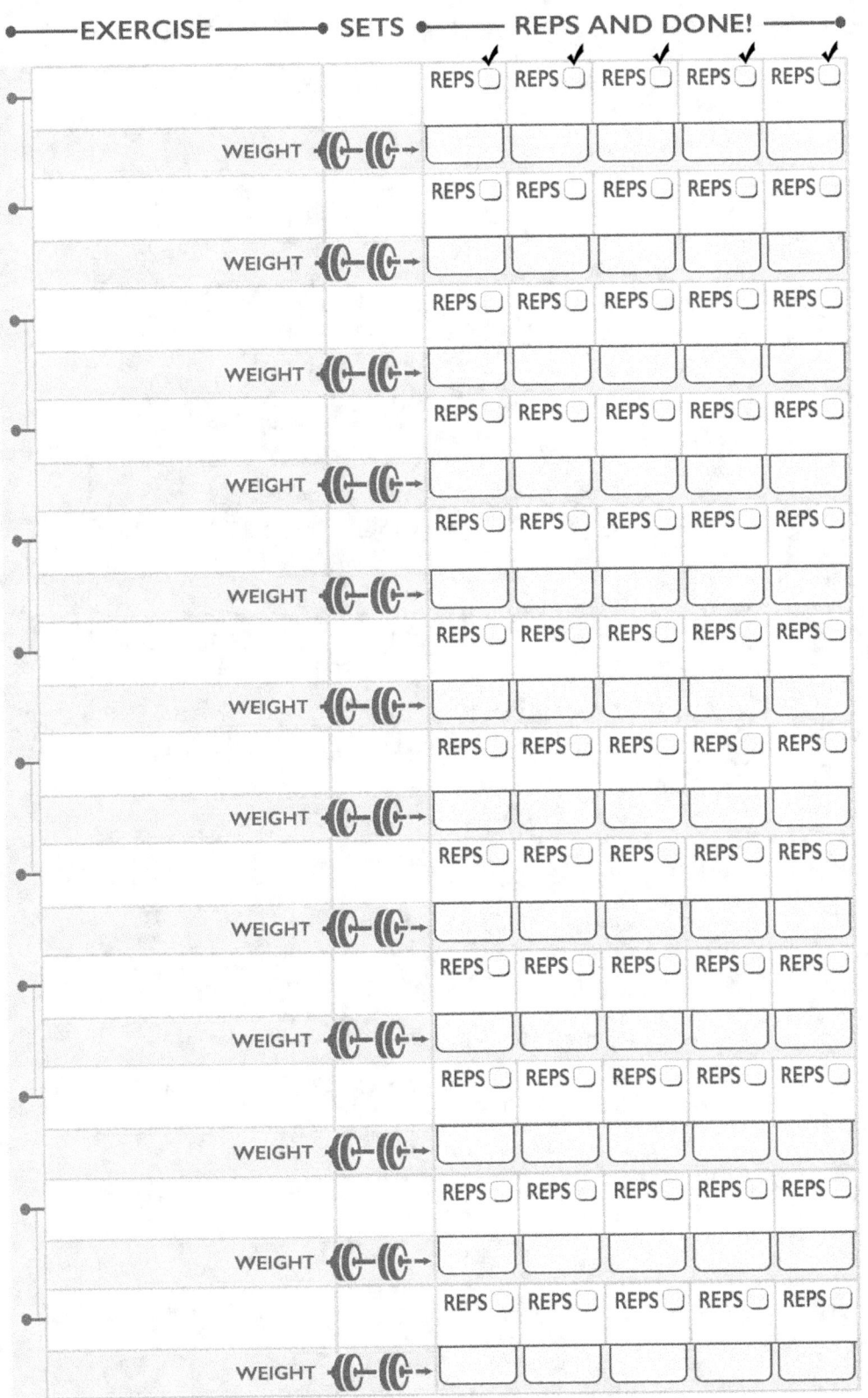

EXERCISE	SETS	REPS	REPS	REPS	REPS
	WEIGHT				
		REPS	REPS	REPS	REPS
	WEIGHT				
		REPS	REPS	REPS	REPS
	WEIGHT				
		REPS	REPS	REPS	REPS
	WEIGHT				
		REPS	REPS	REPS	REPS
	WEIGHT				
		REPS	REPS	REPS	REPS
	WEIGHT				
		REPS	REPS	REPS	REPS
	WEIGHT				
		REPS	REPS	REPS	REPS
	WEIGHT				
		REPS	REPS	REPS	REPS
	WEIGHT				
		REPS	REPS	REPS	REPS
	WEIGHT				

EXERCISE	SETS	REPS AND DONE!				
		REPS ☑	REPS ☑	REPS ☑	REPS ☑	REPS ☑
	WEIGHT					
		REPS ☐	REPS ☐	REPS ☐	REPS ☐	REPS ☐
	WEIGHT					
		REPS ☐	REPS ☐	REPS ☐	REPS ☐	REPS ☐
	WEIGHT					
		REPS ☐	REPS ☐	REPS ☐	REPS ☐	REPS ☐
	WEIGHT					
		REPS ☐	REPS ☐	REPS ☐	REPS ☐	REPS ☐
	WEIGHT					
		REPS ☐	REPS ☐	REPS ☐	REPS ☐	REPS ☐
	WEIGHT					
		REPS ☐	REPS ☐	REPS ☐	REPS ☐	REPS ☐
	WEIGHT					
		REPS ☐	REPS ☐	REPS ☐	REPS ☐	REPS ☐
	WEIGHT					
		REPS ☐	REPS ☐	REPS ☐	REPS ☐	REPS ☐
	WEIGHT					
		REPS ☐	REPS ☐	REPS ☐	REPS ☐	REPS ☐
	WEIGHT					

EXERCISE	SETS	REPS AND DONE! ✓ ✓ ✓ ✓			
		REPS ☐	REPS ☐	REPS ☐	REPS ☐
	WEIGHT ◖€–€◗→				
		REPS ☐	REPS ☐	REPS ☐	REPS ☐
	WEIGHT ◖€–€◗→				
		REPS ☐	REPS ☐	REPS ☐	REPS ☐
	WEIGHT ◖€–€◗→				
		REPS ☐	REPS ☐	REPS ☐	REPS ☐
	WEIGHT ◖€–€◗→				
		REPS ☐	REPS ☐	REPS ☐	REPS ☐
	WEIGHT ◖€–€◗→				
		REPS ☐	REPS ☐	REPS ☐	REPS ☐
	WEIGHT ◖€–€◗→				
		REPS ☐	REPS ☐	REPS ☐	REPS ☐
	WEIGHT ◖€–€◗→				
		REPS ☐	REPS ☐	REPS ☐	REPS ☐
	WEIGHT ◖€–€◗→				
		REPS ☐	REPS ☐	REPS ☐	REPS ☐
	WEIGHT ◖€–€◗→				
		REPS ☐	REPS ☐	REPS ☐	REPS ☐
	WEIGHT ◖€–€◗→				

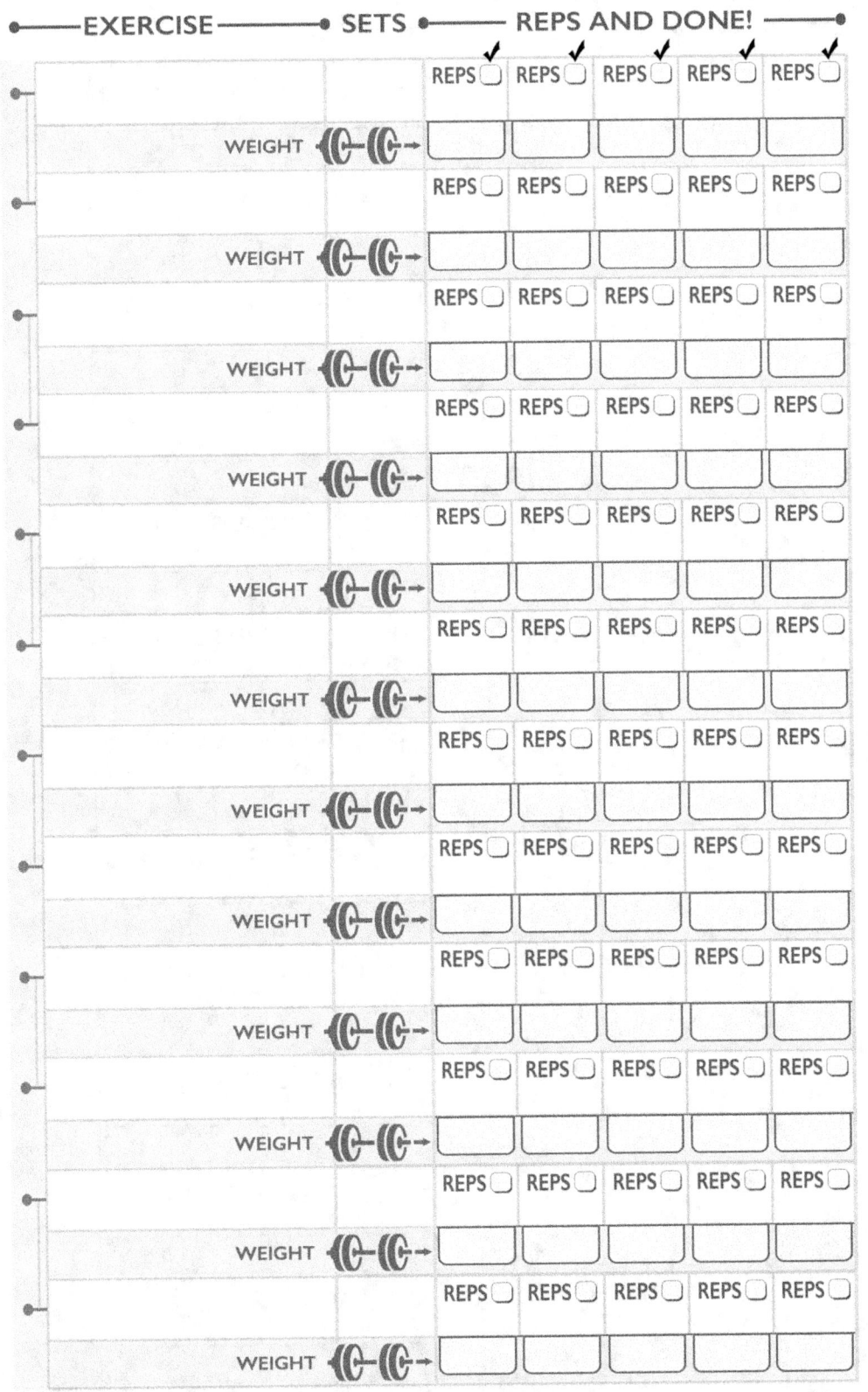

EXERCISE	SETS	REPS AND DONE!			
		REPS ☐	REPS ☐	REPS ☐	REPS ☐
WEIGHT					
		REPS ☐	REPS ☐	REPS ☐	REPS ☐
WEIGHT					
		REPS ☐	REPS ☐	REPS ☐	REPS ☐
WEIGHT					
		REPS ☐	REPS ☐	REPS ☐	REPS ☐
WEIGHT					
		REPS ☐	REPS ☐	REPS ☐	REPS ☐
WEIGHT					
		REPS ☐	REPS ☐	REPS ☐	REPS ☐
WEIGHT					
		REPS ☐	REPS ☐	REPS ☐	REPS ☐
WEIGHT					
		REPS ☐	REPS ☐	REPS ☐	REPS ☐
WEIGHT					
		REPS ☐	REPS ☐	REPS ☐	REPS ☐
WEIGHT					
		REPS ☐	REPS ☐	REPS ☐	REPS ☐
WEIGHT					
		REPS ☐	REPS ☐	REPS ☐	REPS ☐
WEIGHT					

EXERCISE	SETS	REPS AND DONE!				
		REPS ☐	REPS ☐	REPS ☐	REPS ☐	REPS ☐
	WEIGHT ◀⬤-⬤▶					
		REPS ☐	REPS ☐	REPS ☐	REPS ☐	REPS ☐
	WEIGHT ◀⬤-⬤▶					
		REPS ☐	REPS ☐	REPS ☐	REPS ☐	REPS ☐
	WEIGHT ◀⬤-⬤▶					
		REPS ☐	REPS ☐	REPS ☐	REPS ☐	REPS ☐
	WEIGHT ◀⬤-⬤▶					
		REPS ☐	REPS ☐	REPS ☐	REPS ☐	REPS ☐
	WEIGHT ◀⬤-⬤▶					
		REPS ☐	REPS ☐	REPS ☐	REPS ☐	REPS ☐
	WEIGHT ◀⬤-⬤▶					
		REPS ☐	REPS ☐	REPS ☐	REPS ☐	REPS ☐
	WEIGHT ◀⬤-⬤▶					
		REPS ☐	REPS ☐	REPS ☐	REPS ☐	REPS ☐
	WEIGHT ◀⬤-⬤▶					
		REPS ☐	REPS ☐	REPS ☐	REPS ☐	REPS ☐
	WEIGHT ◀⬤-⬤▶					
		REPS ☐	REPS ☐	REPS ☐	REPS ☐	REPS ☐
	WEIGHT ◀⬤-⬤▶					
		REPS ☐	REPS ☐	REPS ☐	REPS ☐	REPS ☐
	WEIGHT ◀⬤-⬤▶					

EXERCISE	SETS	REPS	REPS	REPS	REPS
	WEIGHT				
		REPS	REPS	REPS	REPS
	WEIGHT				
		REPS	REPS	REPS	REPS
	WEIGHT				
		REPS	REPS	REPS	REPS
	WEIGHT				
		REPS	REPS	REPS	REPS
	WEIGHT				
		REPS	REPS	REPS	REPS
	WEIGHT				
		REPS	REPS	REPS	REPS
	WEIGHT				
		REPS	REPS	REPS	REPS
	WEIGHT				
		REPS	REPS	REPS	REPS
	WEIGHT				
		REPS	REPS	REPS	REPS
	WEIGHT				
		REPS	REPS	REPS	REPS
	WEIGHT				

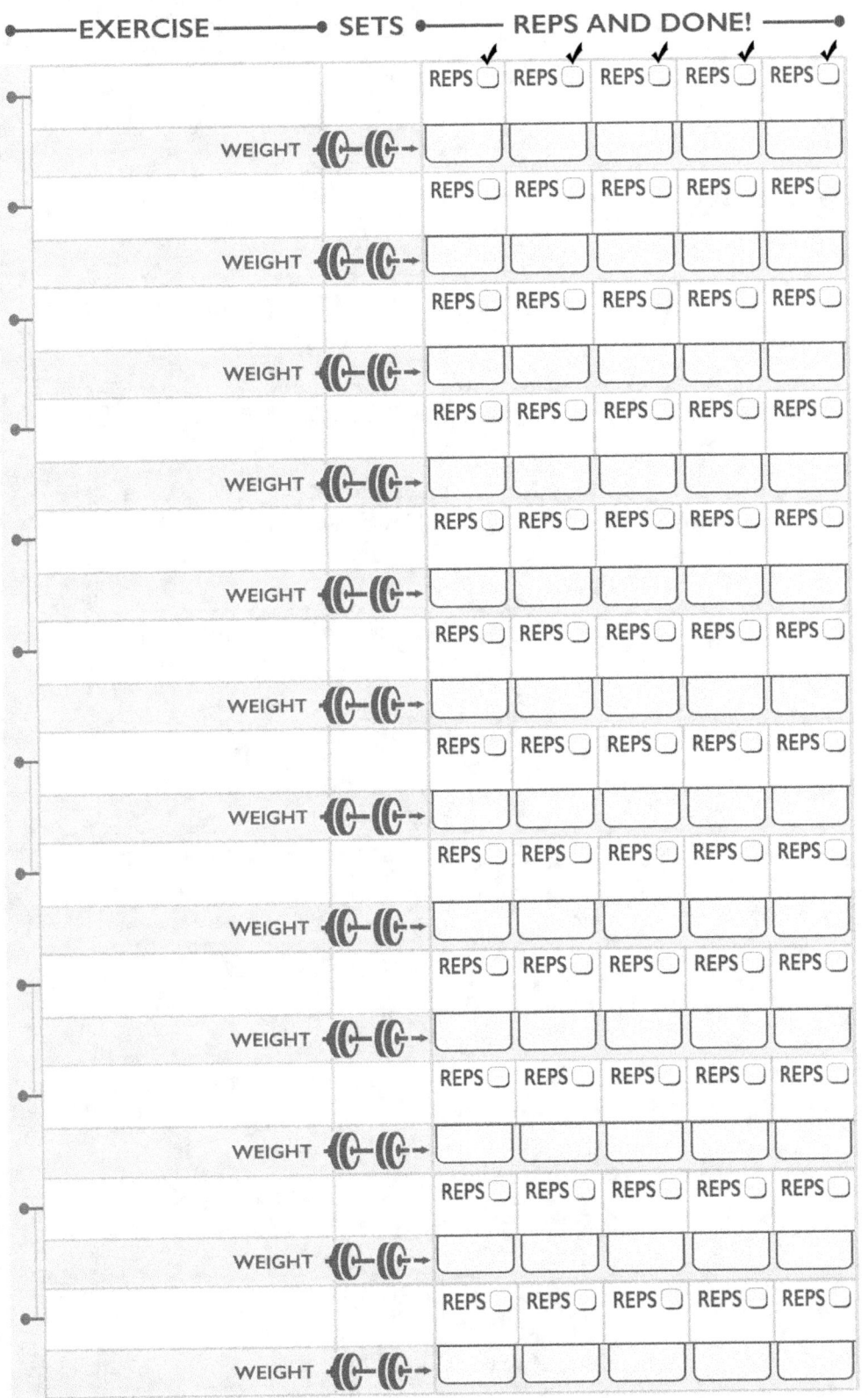

EXERCISE	SETS	REPS	REPS	REPS	REPS
	WEIGHT				
		REPS	REPS	REPS	REPS
	WEIGHT				
		REPS	REPS	REPS	REPS
	WEIGHT				
		REPS	REPS	REPS	REPS
	WEIGHT				
		REPS	REPS	REPS	REPS
	WEIGHT				
		REPS	REPS	REPS	REPS
	WEIGHT				
		REPS	REPS	REPS	REPS
	WEIGHT				
		REPS	REPS	REPS	REPS
	WEIGHT				
		REPS	REPS	REPS	REPS
	WEIGHT				
		REPS	REPS	REPS	REPS
	WEIGHT				
		REPS	REPS	REPS	REPS
	WEIGHT				

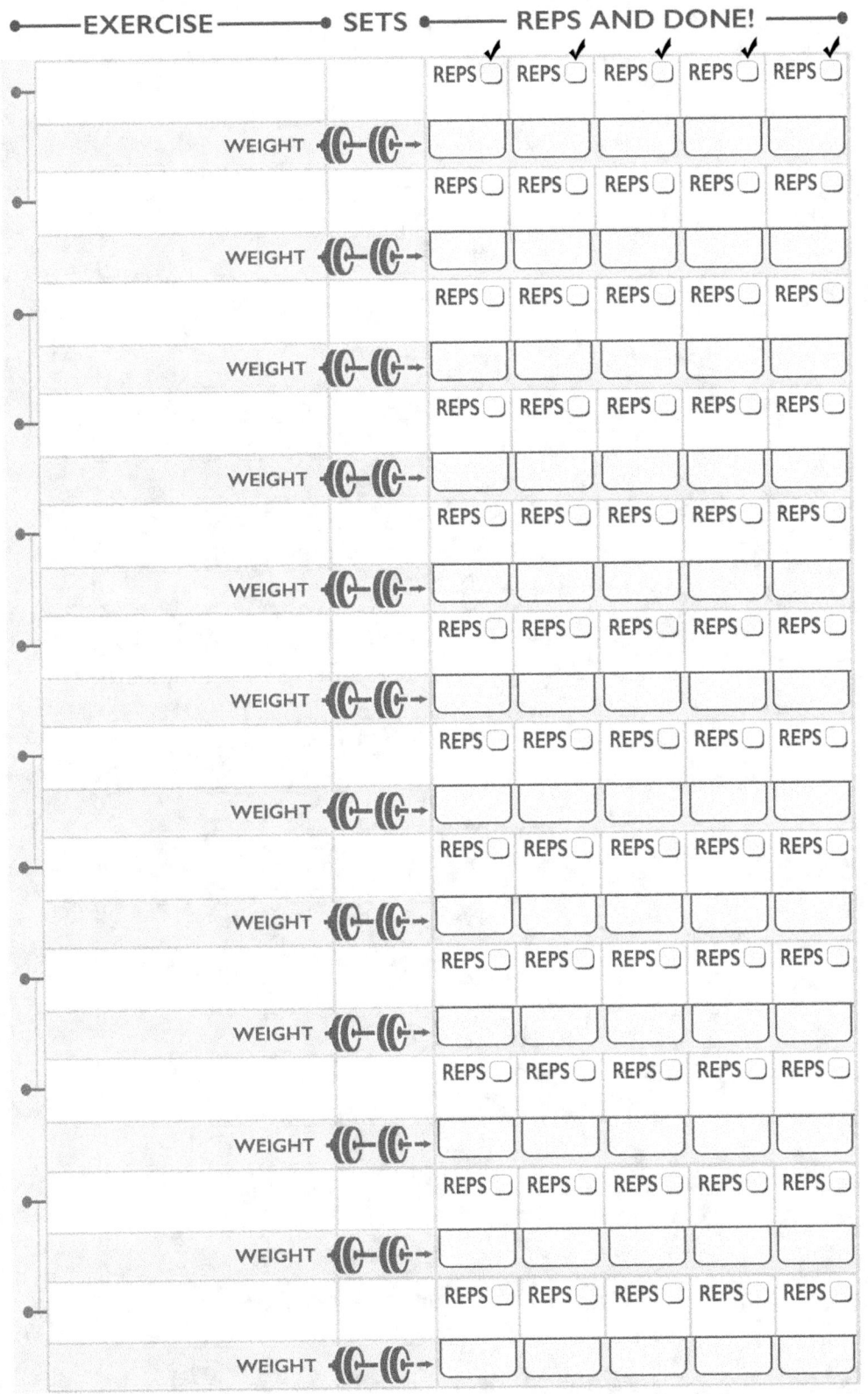

EXERCISE	SETS	REPS	REPS	REPS	REPS
WEIGHT					
		REPS	REPS	REPS	REPS
WEIGHT					
		REPS	REPS	REPS	REPS
WEIGHT					
		REPS	REPS	REPS	REPS
WEIGHT					
		REPS	REPS	REPS	REPS
WEIGHT					
		REPS	REPS	REPS	REPS
WEIGHT					
		REPS	REPS	REPS	REPS
WEIGHT					
		REPS	REPS	REPS	REPS
WEIGHT					
		REPS	REPS	REPS	REPS
WEIGHT					
		REPS	REPS	REPS	REPS
WEIGHT					

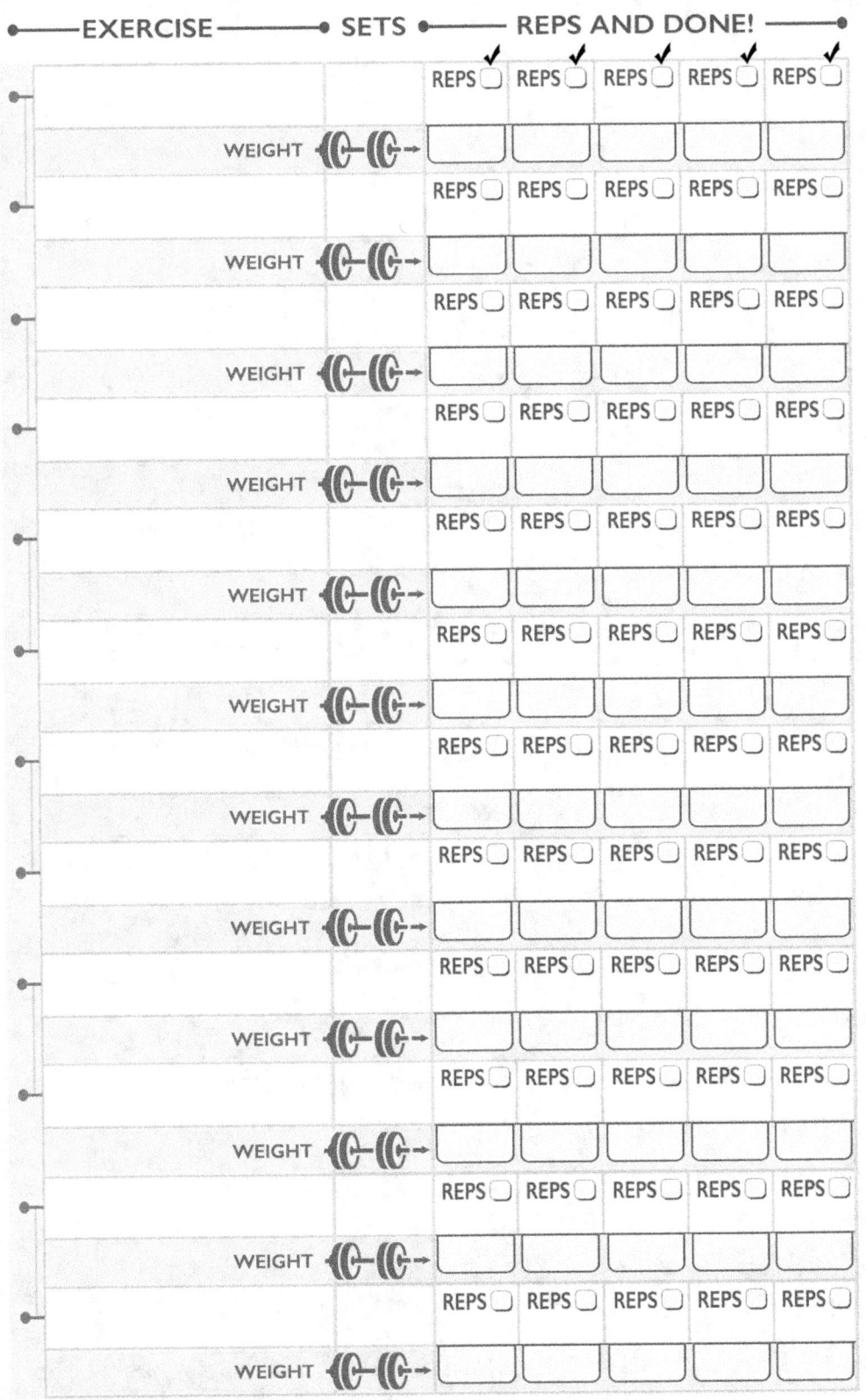

EXERCISE	SETS	REPS ✔	REPS ✔	REPS ✔	REPS ✔
	WEIGHT				
		REPS	REPS	REPS	REPS
	WEIGHT				
		REPS	REPS	REPS	REPS
	WEIGHT				
		REPS	REPS	REPS	REPS
	WEIGHT				
		REPS	REPS	REPS	REPS
	WEIGHT				
		REPS	REPS	REPS	REPS
	WEIGHT				
		REPS	REPS	REPS	REPS
	WEIGHT				
		REPS	REPS	REPS	REPS
	WEIGHT				
		REPS	REPS	REPS	REPS
	WEIGHT				
		REPS	REPS	REPS	REPS
	WEIGHT				

EXERCISE	SETS	REPS AND DONE!				
		REPS ☐	REPS ☐	REPS ☐	REPS ☐	REPS ☐
WEIGHT						
		REPS ☐	REPS ☐	REPS ☐	REPS ☐	REPS ☐
WEIGHT						
		REPS ☐	REPS ☐	REPS ☐	REPS ☐	REPS ☐
WEIGHT						
		REPS ☐	REPS ☐	REPS ☐	REPS ☐	REPS ☐
WEIGHT						
		REPS ☐	REPS ☐	REPS ☐	REPS ☐	REPS ☐
WEIGHT						
		REPS ☐	REPS ☐	REPS ☐	REPS ☐	REPS ☐
WEIGHT						
		REPS ☐	REPS ☐	REPS ☐	REPS ☐	REPS ☐
WEIGHT						
		REPS ☐	REPS ☐	REPS ☐	REPS ☐	REPS ☐
WEIGHT						
		REPS ☐	REPS ☐	REPS ☐	REPS ☐	REPS ☐
WEIGHT						
		REPS ☐	REPS ☐	REPS ☐	REPS ☐	REPS ☐
WEIGHT						

EXERCISE	SETS	REPS ✓	REPS ✓	REPS ✓	REPS ✓
	WEIGHT				
		REPS	REPS	REPS	REPS
	WEIGHT				
		REPS	REPS	REPS	REPS
	WEIGHT				
		REPS	REPS	REPS	REPS
	WEIGHT				
		REPS	REPS	REPS	REPS
	WEIGHT				
		REPS	REPS	REPS	REPS
	WEIGHT				
		REPS	REPS	REPS	REPS
	WEIGHT				
		REPS	REPS	REPS	REPS
	WEIGHT				
		REPS	REPS	REPS	REPS
	WEIGHT				
		REPS	REPS	REPS	REPS
	WEIGHT				

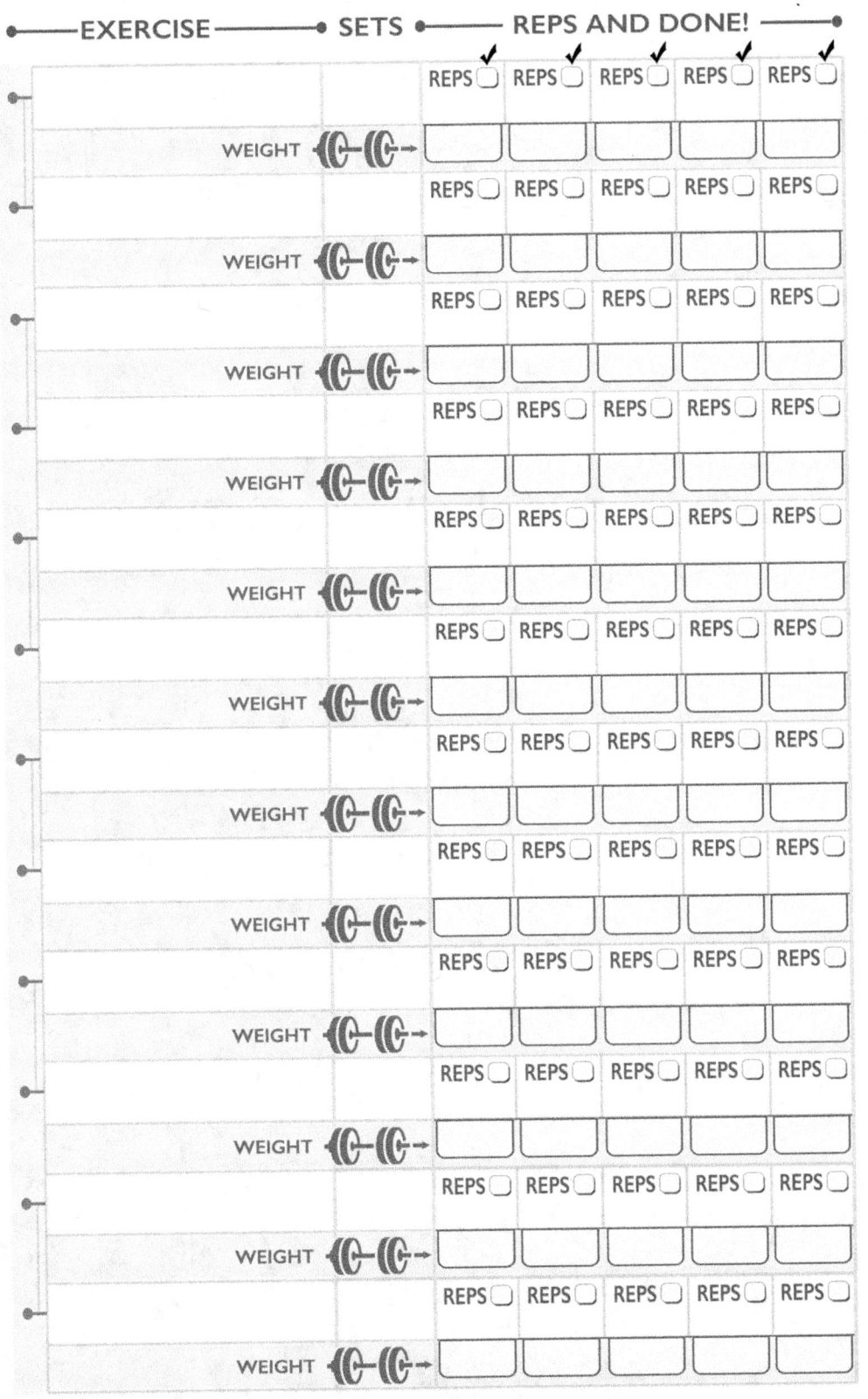

EXERCISE	SETS	REPS AND DONE!			
		REPS ☐	REPS ☐	REPS ☐	REPS ☐
	WEIGHT				
		REPS ☐	REPS ☐	REPS ☐	REPS ☐
	WEIGHT				
		REPS ☐	REPS ☐	REPS ☐	REPS ☐
	WEIGHT				
		REPS ☐	REPS ☐	REPS ☐	REPS ☐
	WEIGHT				
		REPS ☐	REPS ☐	REPS ☐	REPS ☐
	WEIGHT				
		REPS ☐	REPS ☐	REPS ☐	REPS ☐
	WEIGHT				
		REPS ☐	REPS ☐	REPS ☐	REPS ☐
	WEIGHT				
		REPS ☐	REPS ☐	REPS ☐	REPS ☐
	WEIGHT				
		REPS ☐	REPS ☐	REPS ☐	REPS ☐
	WEIGHT				
		REPS ☐	REPS ☐	REPS ☐	REPS ☐
	WEIGHT				
		REPS ☐	REPS ☐	REPS ☐	REPS ☐
	WEIGHT				

EXERCISE	SETS	REPS AND DONE!				
		REPS ☐	REPS ☐	REPS ☐	REPS ☐	REPS ☐
	WEIGHT					
		REPS ☐	REPS ☐	REPS ☐	REPS ☐	REPS ☐
	WEIGHT					
		REPS ☐	REPS ☐	REPS ☐	REPS ☐	REPS ☐
	WEIGHT					
		REPS ☐	REPS ☐	REPS ☐	REPS ☐	REPS ☐
	WEIGHT					
		REPS ☐	REPS ☐	REPS ☐	REPS ☐	REPS ☐
	WEIGHT					
		REPS ☐	REPS ☐	REPS ☐	REPS ☐	REPS ☐
	WEIGHT					
		REPS ☐	REPS ☐	REPS ☐	REPS ☐	REPS ☐
	WEIGHT					
		REPS ☐	REPS ☐	REPS ☐	REPS ☐	REPS ☐
	WEIGHT					
		REPS ☐	REPS ☐	REPS ☐	REPS ☐	REPS ☐
	WEIGHT					
		REPS ☐	REPS ☐	REPS ☐	REPS ☐	REPS ☐
	WEIGHT					
		REPS ☐	REPS ☐	REPS ☐	REPS ☐	REPS ☐
	WEIGHT					

EXERCISE	SETS	REPS AND DONE!			
		REPS ☐	REPS ☐	REPS ☐	REPS ☐
WEIGHT					
		REPS ☐	REPS ☐	REPS ☐	REPS ☐
WEIGHT					
		REPS ☐	REPS ☐	REPS ☐	REPS ☐
WEIGHT					
		REPS ☐	REPS ☐	REPS ☐	REPS ☐
WEIGHT					
		REPS ☐	REPS ☐	REPS ☐	REPS ☐
WEIGHT					
		REPS ☐	REPS ☐	REPS ☐	REPS ☐
WEIGHT					
		REPS ☐	REPS ☐	REPS ☐	REPS ☐
WEIGHT					
		REPS ☐	REPS ☐	REPS ☐	REPS ☐
WEIGHT					
		REPS ☐	REPS ☐	REPS ☐	REPS ☐
WEIGHT					
		REPS ☐	REPS ☐	REPS ☐	REPS ☐
WEIGHT					

EXERCISE	SETS	REPS AND DONE!				
		REPS ☐	REPS ☐	REPS ☐	REPS ☐	REPS ☐
	WEIGHT					
		REPS ☐	REPS ☐	REPS ☐	REPS ☐	REPS ☐
	WEIGHT					
		REPS ☐	REPS ☐	REPS ☐	REPS ☐	REPS ☐
	WEIGHT					
		REPS ☐	REPS ☐	REPS ☐	REPS ☐	REPS ☐
	WEIGHT					
		REPS ☐	REPS ☐	REPS ☐	REPS ☐	REPS ☐
	WEIGHT					
		REPS ☐	REPS ☐	REPS ☐	REPS ☐	REPS ☐
	WEIGHT					
		REPS ☐	REPS ☐	REPS ☐	REPS ☐	REPS ☐
	WEIGHT					
		REPS ☐	REPS ☐	REPS ☐	REPS ☐	REPS ☐
	WEIGHT					
		REPS ☐	REPS ☐	REPS ☐	REPS ☐	REPS ☐
	WEIGHT					
		REPS ☐	REPS ☐	REPS ☐	REPS ☐	REPS ☐
	WEIGHT					
		REPS ☐	REPS ☐	REPS ☐	REPS ☐	REPS ☐
	WEIGHT					

EXERCISE	SETS	REPS ✓	REPS ✓	REPS ✓	REPS ✓
	WEIGHT				
		REPS	REPS	REPS	REPS
	WEIGHT				
		REPS	REPS	REPS	REPS
	WEIGHT				
		REPS	REPS	REPS	REPS
	WEIGHT				
		REPS	REPS	REPS	REPS
	WEIGHT				
		REPS	REPS	REPS	REPS
	WEIGHT				
		REPS	REPS	REPS	REPS
	WEIGHT				
		REPS	REPS	REPS	REPS
	WEIGHT				
		REPS	REPS	REPS	REPS
	WEIGHT				
		REPS	REPS	REPS	REPS
	WEIGHT				
		REPS	REPS	REPS	REPS
	WEIGHT				

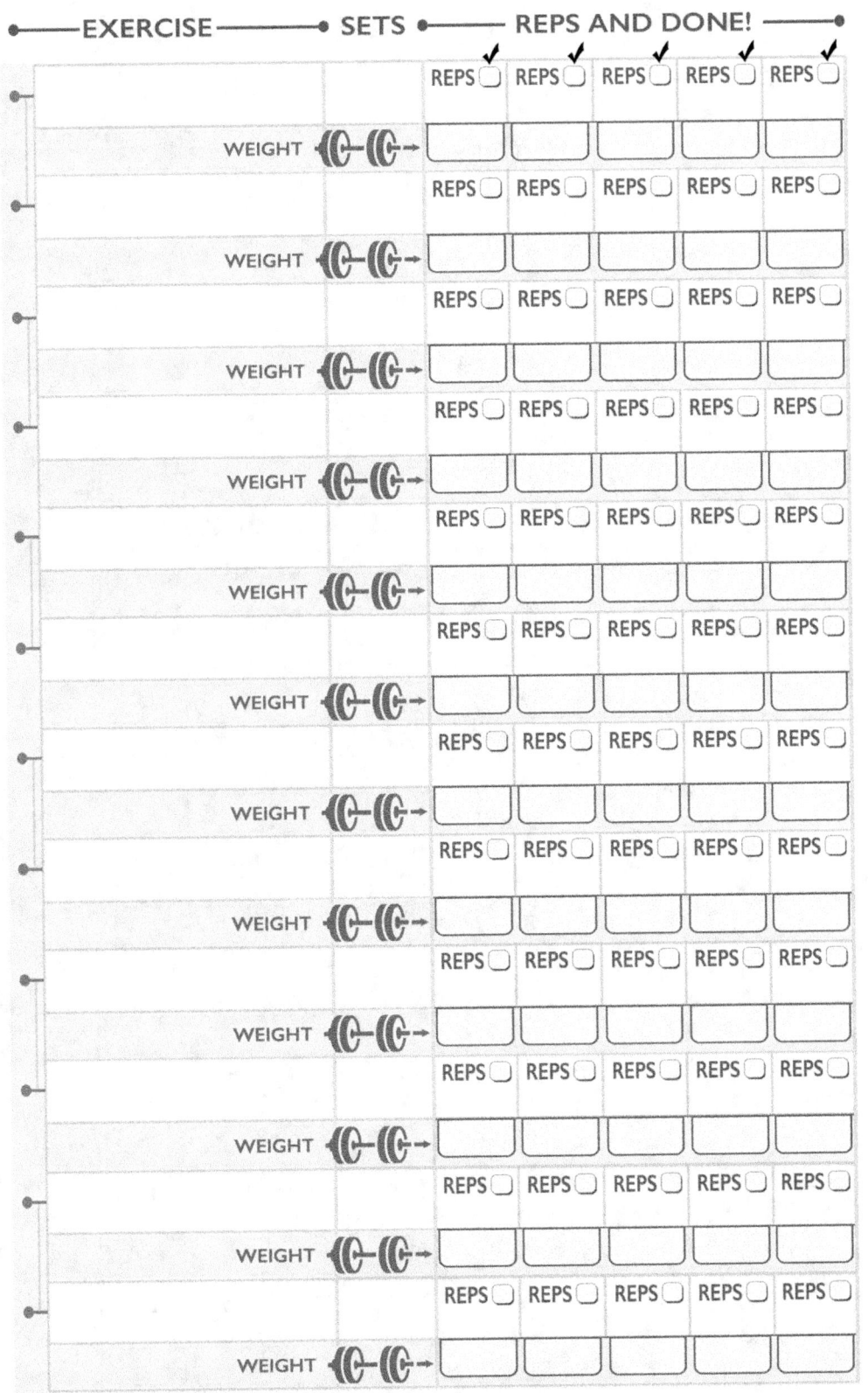

		REPS ☐	REPS ☐	REPS ☐	REPS ☐
	WEIGHT ◀▣–▣▶				
		REPS ☐	REPS ☐	REPS ☐	REPS ☐
	WEIGHT ◀▣–▣▶				
		REPS ☐	REPS ☐	REPS ☐	REPS ☐
	WEIGHT ◀▣–▣▶				
		REPS ☐	REPS ☐	REPS ☐	REPS ☐
	WEIGHT ◀▣–▣▶				
		REPS ☐	REPS ☐	REPS ☐	REPS ☐
	WEIGHT ◀▣–▣▶				
		REPS ☐	REPS ☐	REPS ☐	REPS ☐
	WEIGHT ◀▣–▣▶				
		REPS ☐	REPS ☐	REPS ☐	REPS ☐
	WEIGHT ◀▣–▣▶				
		REPS ☐	REPS ☐	REPS ☐	REPS ☐
	WEIGHT ◀▣–▣▶				
		REPS ☐	REPS ☐	REPS ☐	REPS ☐
	WEIGHT ◀▣–▣▶				
		REPS ☐	REPS ☐	REPS ☐	REPS ☐
	WEIGHT ◀▣–▣▶				

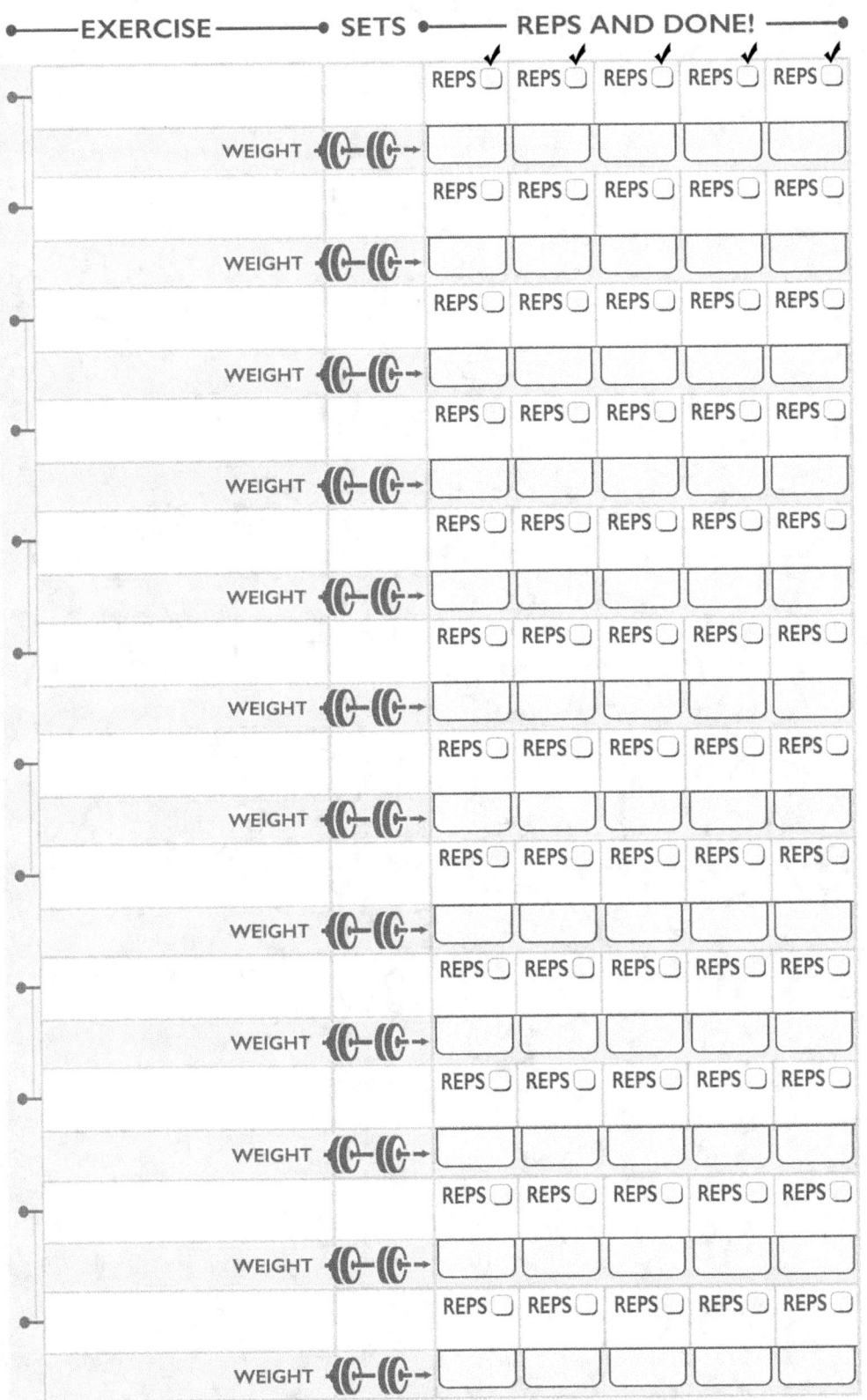

EXERCISE	SETS	REPS AND DONE!			
		REPS ☐	REPS ☐	REPS ☐	REPS ☐
WEIGHT					
		REPS ☐	REPS ☐	REPS ☐	REPS ☐
WEIGHT					
		REPS ☐	REPS ☐	REPS ☐	REPS ☐
WEIGHT					
		REPS ☐	REPS ☐	REPS ☐	REPS ☐
WEIGHT					
		REPS ☐	REPS ☐	REPS ☐	REPS ☐
WEIGHT					
		REPS ☐	REPS ☐	REPS ☐	REPS ☐
WEIGHT					
		REPS ☐	REPS ☐	REPS ☐	REPS ☐
WEIGHT					
		REPS ☐	REPS ☐	REPS ☐	REPS ☐
WEIGHT					
		REPS ☐	REPS ☐	REPS ☐	REPS ☐
WEIGHT					
		REPS ☐	REPS ☐	REPS ☐	REPS ☐
WEIGHT					

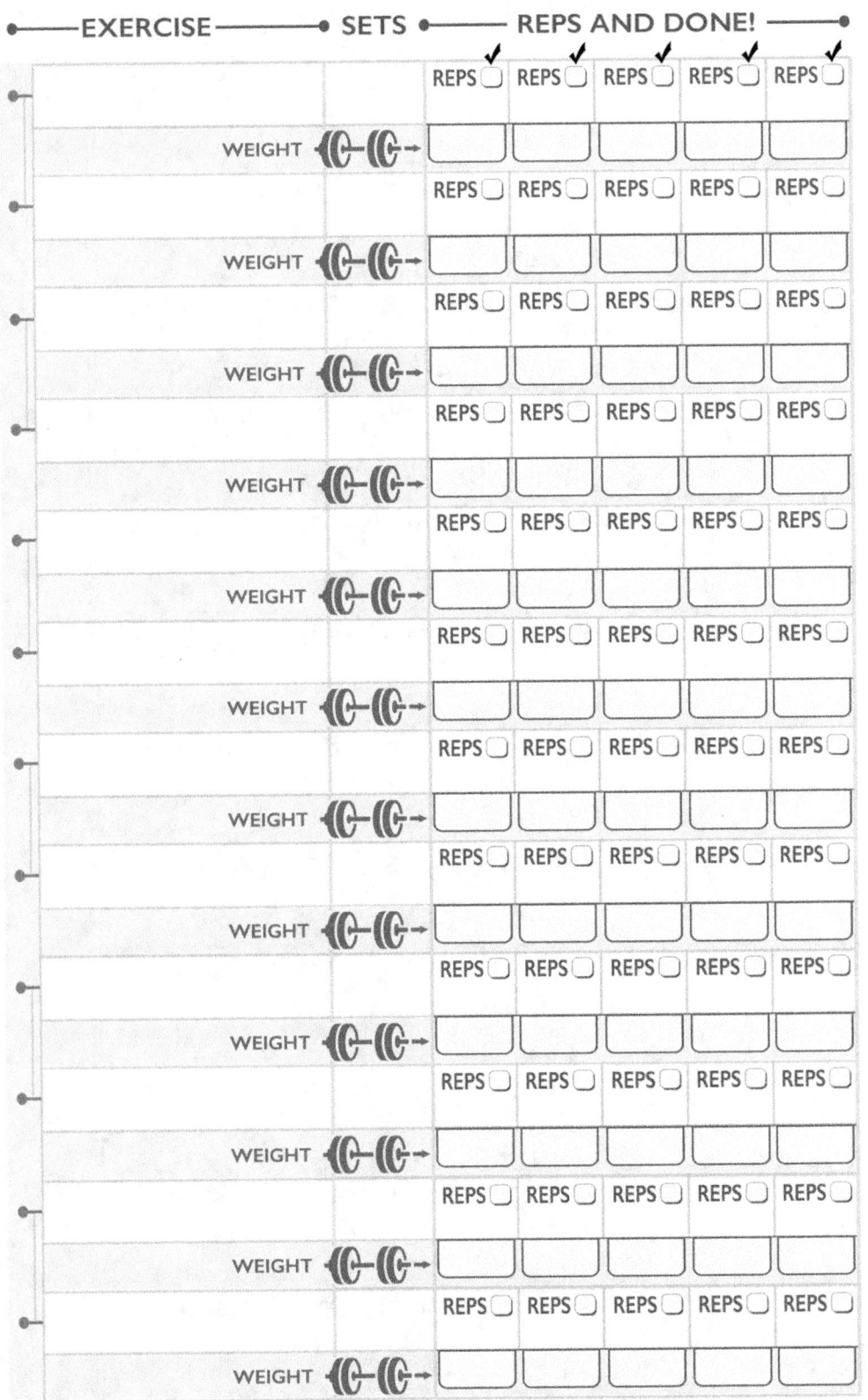

EXERCISE	SETS	REPS AND DONE!			
		REPS ☐	REPS ☐	REPS ☐	REPS ☐
	WEIGHT				
		REPS ☐	REPS ☐	REPS ☐	REPS ☐
	WEIGHT				
		REPS ☐	REPS ☐	REPS ☐	REPS ☐
	WEIGHT				
		REPS ☐	REPS ☐	REPS ☐	REPS ☐
	WEIGHT				
		REPS ☐	REPS ☐	REPS ☐	REPS ☐
	WEIGHT				
		REPS ☐	REPS ☐	REPS ☐	REPS ☐
	WEIGHT				
		REPS ☐	REPS ☐	REPS ☐	REPS ☐
	WEIGHT				
		REPS ☐	REPS ☐	REPS ☐	REPS ☐
	WEIGHT				
		REPS ☐	REPS ☐	REPS ☐	REPS ☐
	WEIGHT				
		REPS ☐	REPS ☐	REPS ☐	REPS ☐
	WEIGHT				
		REPS ☐	REPS ☐	REPS ☐	REPS ☐
	WEIGHT				

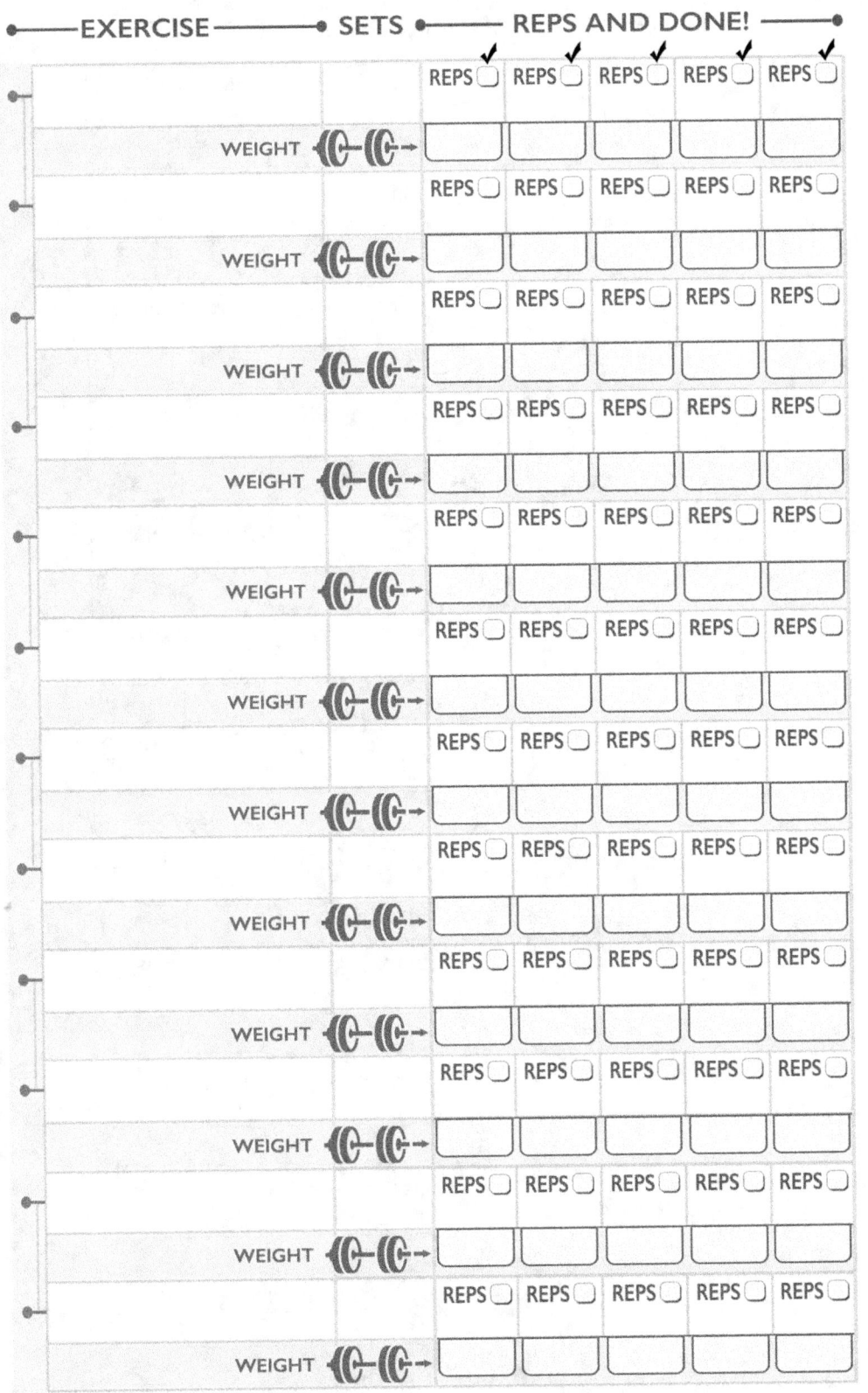

		REPS ☐	REPS ☐	REPS ☐	REPS ☐
WEIGHT					
		REPS ☐	REPS ☐	REPS ☐	REPS ☐
WEIGHT					
		REPS ☐	REPS ☐	REPS ☐	REPS ☐
WEIGHT					
		REPS ☐	REPS ☐	REPS ☐	REPS ☐
WEIGHT					
		REPS ☐	REPS ☐	REPS ☐	REPS ☐
WEIGHT					
		REPS ☐	REPS ☐	REPS ☐	REPS ☐
WEIGHT					
		REPS ☐	REPS ☐	REPS ☐	REPS ☐
WEIGHT					
		REPS ☐	REPS ☐	REPS ☐	REPS ☐
WEIGHT					
		REPS ☐	REPS ☐	REPS ☐	REPS ☐
WEIGHT					
		REPS ☐	REPS ☐	REPS ☐	REPS ☐
WEIGHT					
		REPS ☐	REPS ☐	REPS ☐	REPS ☐
WEIGHT					

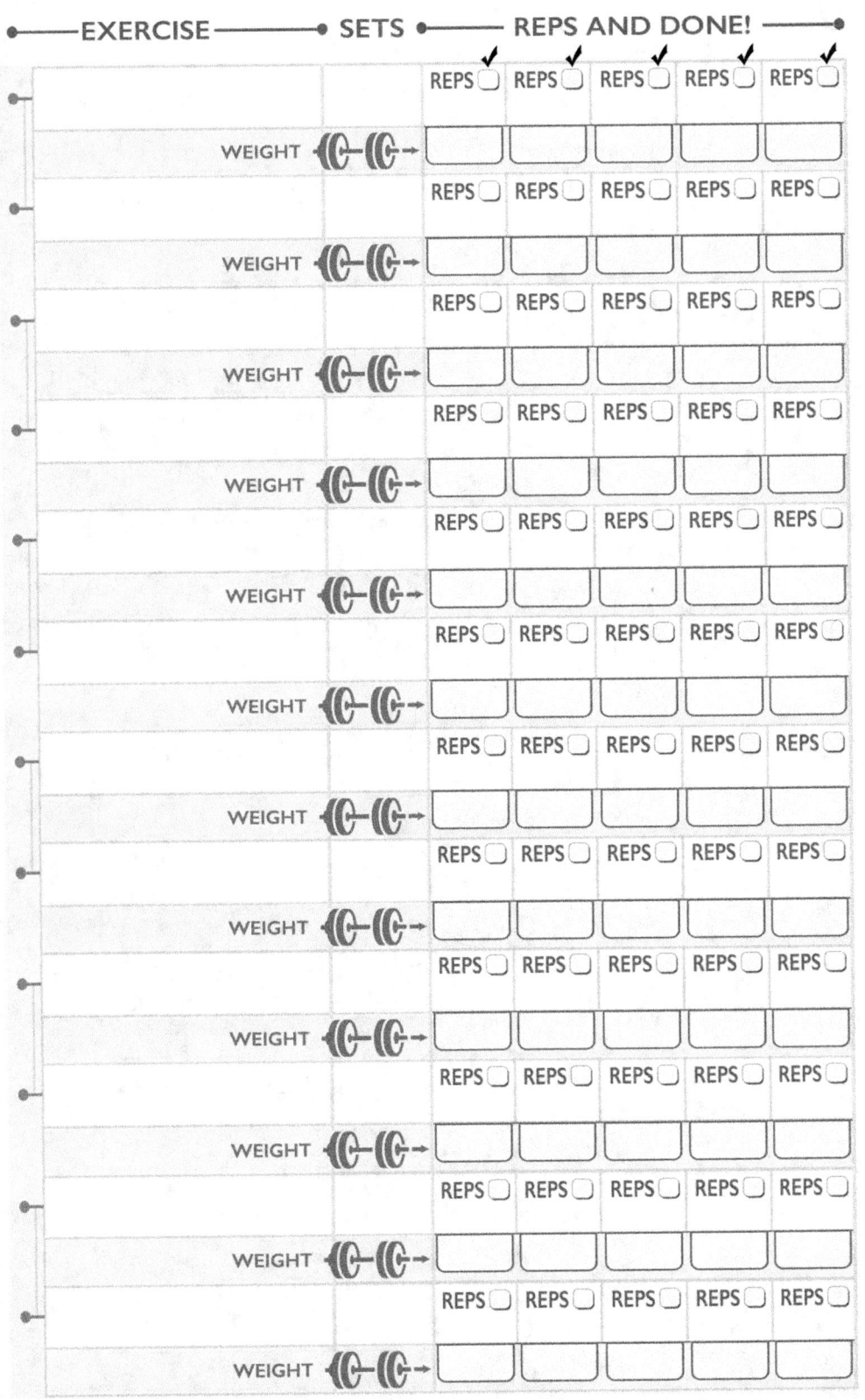

EXERCISE	SETS	REPS AND DONE!			
		REPS ☐	REPS ☐	REPS ☐	REPS ☐
WEIGHT					
		REPS ☐	REPS ☐	REPS ☐	REPS ☐
WEIGHT					
		REPS ☐	REPS ☐	REPS ☐	REPS ☐
WEIGHT					
		REPS ☐	REPS ☐	REPS ☐	REPS ☐
WEIGHT					
		REPS ☐	REPS ☐	REPS ☐	REPS ☐
WEIGHT					
		REPS ☐	REPS ☐	REPS ☐	REPS ☐
WEIGHT					
		REPS ☐	REPS ☐	REPS ☐	REPS ☐
WEIGHT					
		REPS ☐	REPS ☐	REPS ☐	REPS ☐
WEIGHT					
		REPS ☐	REPS ☐	REPS ☐	REPS ☐
WEIGHT					
		REPS ☐	REPS ☐	REPS ☐	REPS ☐
WEIGHT					
		REPS ☐	REPS ☐	REPS ☐	REPS ☐
WEIGHT					

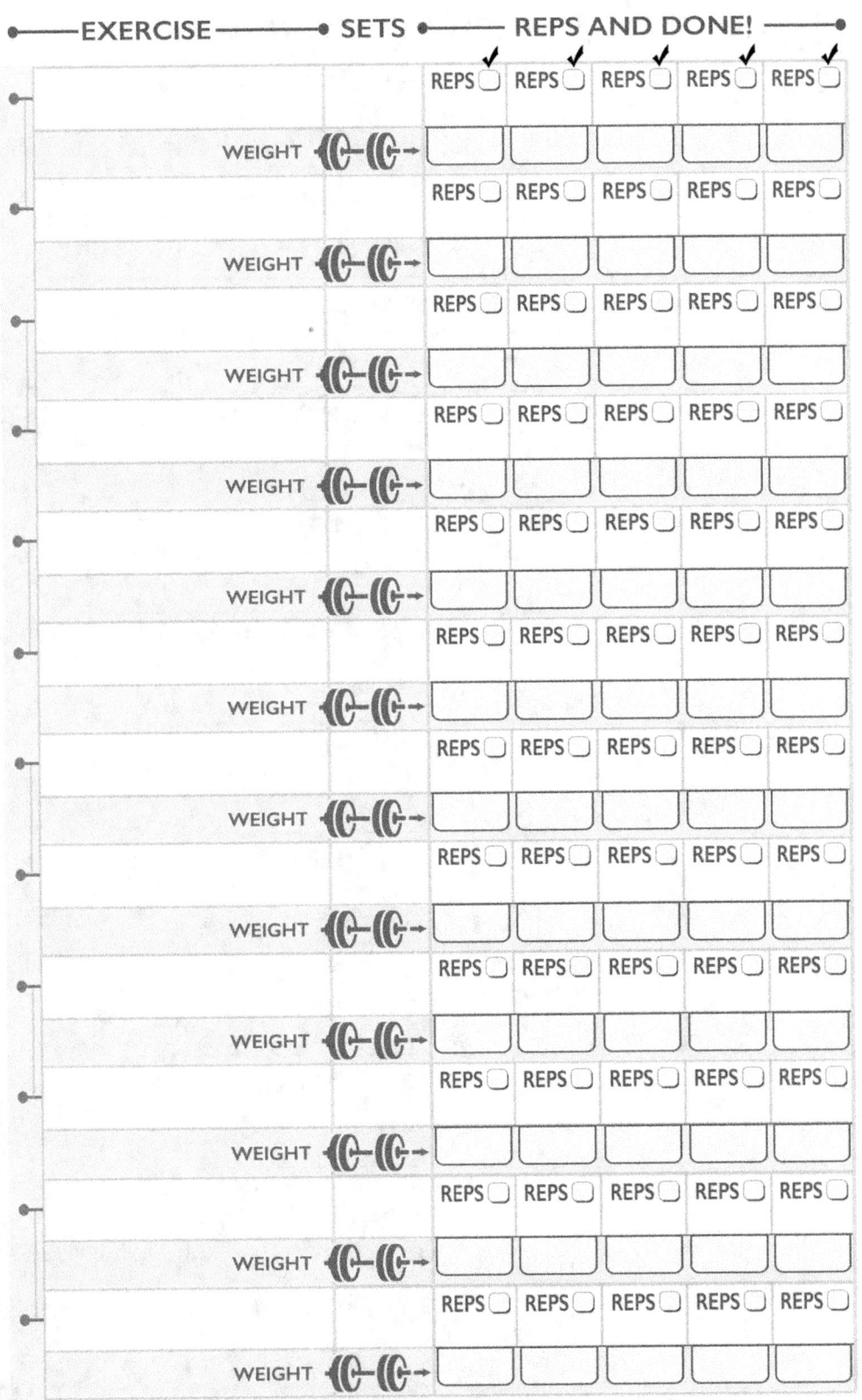

EXERCISE	SETS	REPS	REPS	REPS	REPS
	WEIGHT				
		REPS	REPS	REPS	REPS
	WEIGHT				
		REPS	REPS	REPS	REPS
	WEIGHT				
		REPS	REPS	REPS	REPS
	WEIGHT				
		REPS	REPS	REPS	REPS
	WEIGHT				
		REPS	REPS	REPS	REPS
	WEIGHT				
		REPS	REPS	REPS	REPS
	WEIGHT				
		REPS	REPS	REPS	REPS
	WEIGHT				
		REPS	REPS	REPS	REPS
	WEIGHT				
		REPS	REPS	REPS	REPS
	WEIGHT				
		REPS	REPS	REPS	REPS
	WEIGHT				

		REPS ⬚	REPS ⬚	REPS ⬚	REPS ⬚	REPS ⬚
WEIGHT ◀🏋🏋▶						
		REPS ⬚	REPS ⬚	REPS ⬚	REPS ⬚	REPS ⬚
WEIGHT ◀🏋🏋▶						
		REPS ⬚	REPS ⬚	REPS ⬚	REPS ⬚	REPS ⬚
WEIGHT ◀🏋🏋▶						
		REPS ⬚	REPS ⬚	REPS ⬚	REPS ⬚	REPS ⬚
WEIGHT ◀🏋🏋▶						
		REPS ⬚	REPS ⬚	REPS ⬚	REPS ⬚	REPS ⬚
WEIGHT ◀🏋🏋▶						
		REPS ⬚	REPS ⬚	REPS ⬚	REPS ⬚	REPS ⬚
WEIGHT ◀🏋🏋▶						
		REPS ⬚	REPS ⬚	REPS ⬚	REPS ⬚	REPS ⬚
WEIGHT ◀🏋🏋▶						
		REPS ⬚	REPS ⬚	REPS ⬚	REPS ⬚	REPS ⬚
WEIGHT ◀🏋🏋▶						
		REPS ⬚	REPS ⬚	REPS ⬚	REPS ⬚	REPS ⬚
WEIGHT ◀🏋🏋▶						
		REPS ⬚	REPS ⬚	REPS ⬚	REPS ⬚	REPS ⬚
WEIGHT ◀🏋🏋▶						
		REPS ⬚	REPS ⬚	REPS ⬚	REPS ⬚	REPS ⬚
WEIGHT ◀🏋🏋▶						

EXERCISE	SETS	REPS AND DONE!			
		REPS ☐	REPS ☐	REPS ☐	REPS ☐
WEIGHT 🏋🏋→					
		REPS ☐	REPS ☐	REPS ☐	REPS ☐
WEIGHT 🏋🏋→					
		REPS ☐	REPS ☐	REPS ☐	REPS ☐
WEIGHT 🏋🏋→					
		REPS ☐	REPS ☐	REPS ☐	REPS ☐
WEIGHT 🏋🏋→					
		REPS ☐	REPS ☐	REPS ☐	REPS ☐
WEIGHT 🏋🏋→					
		REPS ☐	REPS ☐	REPS ☐	REPS ☐
WEIGHT 🏋🏋→					
		REPS ☐	REPS ☐	REPS ☐	REPS ☐
WEIGHT 🏋🏋→					
		REPS ☐	REPS ☐	REPS ☐	REPS ☐
WEIGHT 🏋🏋→					
		REPS ☐	REPS ☐	REPS ☐	REPS ☐
WEIGHT 🏋🏋→					
		REPS ☐	REPS ☐	REPS ☐	REPS ☐
WEIGHT 🏋🏋→					
		REPS ☐	REPS ☐	REPS ☐	REPS ☐
WEIGHT 🏋🏋→					

EXERCISE	SETS	REPS ✓	REPS ✓	REPS ✓	REPS ✓	REPS ✓
	WEIGHT					
		REPS ☐	REPS ☐	REPS ☐	REPS ☐	REPS ☐
	WEIGHT					
		REPS ☐	REPS ☐	REPS ☐	REPS ☐	REPS ☐
	WEIGHT					
		REPS ☐	REPS ☐	REPS ☐	REPS ☐	REPS ☐
	WEIGHT					
		REPS ☐	REPS ☐	REPS ☐	REPS ☐	REPS ☐
	WEIGHT					
		REPS ☐	REPS ☐	REPS ☐	REPS ☐	REPS ☐
	WEIGHT					
		REPS ☐	REPS ☐	REPS ☐	REPS ☐	REPS ☐
	WEIGHT					
		REPS ☐	REPS ☐	REPS ☐	REPS ☐	REPS ☐
	WEIGHT					
		REPS ☐	REPS ☐	REPS ☐	REPS ☐	REPS ☐
	WEIGHT					
		REPS ☐	REPS ☐	REPS ☐	REPS ☐	REPS ☐
	WEIGHT					
		REPS ☐	REPS ☐	REPS ☐	REPS ☐	REPS ☐
	WEIGHT					
		REPS ☐	REPS ☐	REPS ☐	REPS ☐	REPS ☐
	WEIGHT					

EXERCISE	SETS	REPS	REPS	REPS	REPS
		REPS ☐	REPS ☐	REPS ☐	REPS ☐
WEIGHT					
		REPS ☐	REPS ☐	REPS ☐	REPS ☐
WEIGHT					
		REPS ☐	REPS ☐	REPS ☐	REPS ☐
WEIGHT					
		REPS ☐	REPS ☐	REPS ☐	REPS ☐
WEIGHT					
		REPS ☐	REPS ☐	REPS ☐	REPS ☐
WEIGHT					
		REPS ☐	REPS ☐	REPS ☐	REPS ☐
WEIGHT					
		REPS ☐	REPS ☐	REPS ☐	REPS ☐
WEIGHT					
		REPS ☐	REPS ☐	REPS ☐	REPS ☐
WEIGHT					
		REPS ☐	REPS ☐	REPS ☐	REPS ☐
WEIGHT					
		REPS ☐	REPS ☐	REPS ☐	REPS ☐
WEIGHT					
		REPS ☐	REPS ☐	REPS ☐	REPS ☐
WEIGHT					

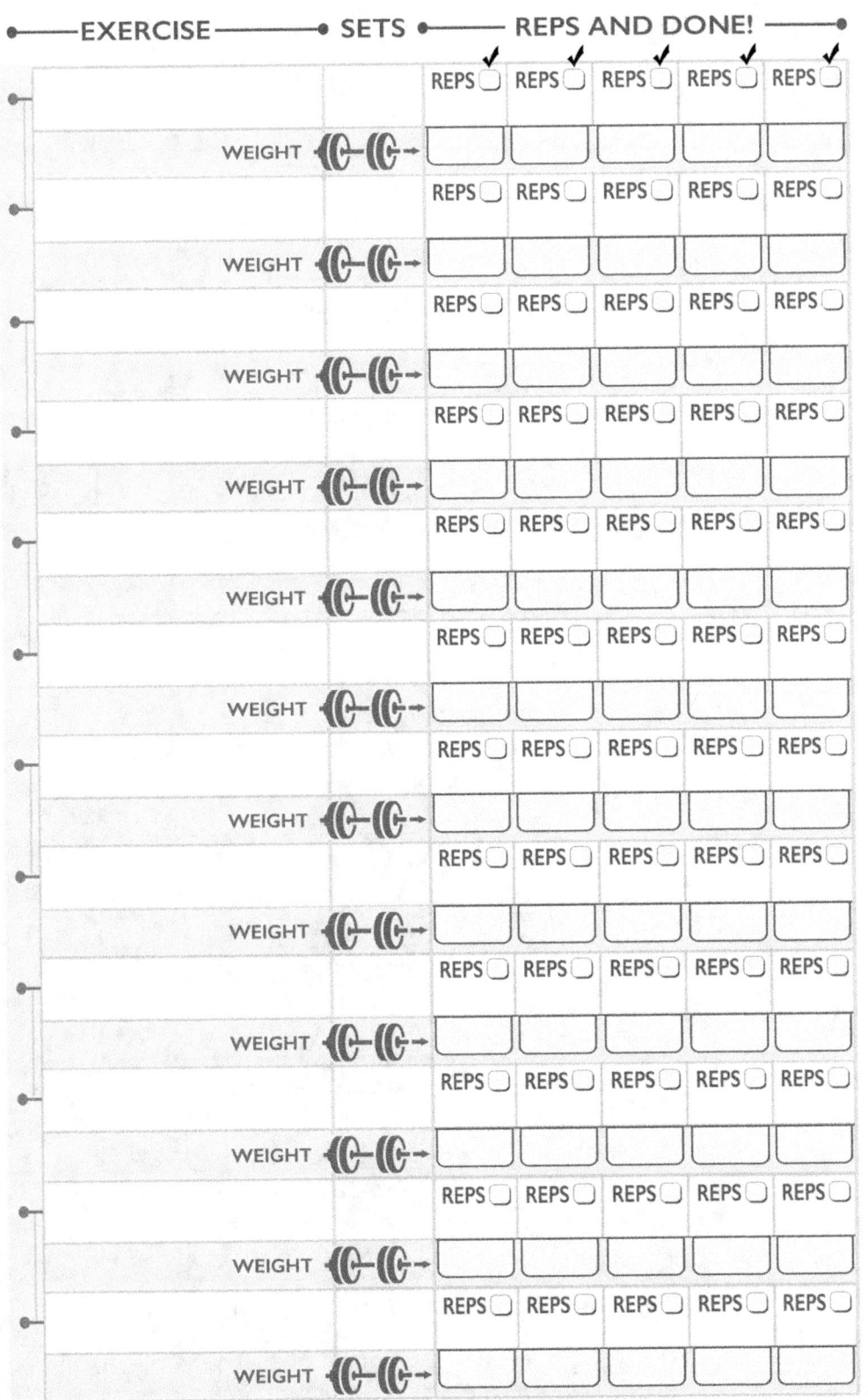

EXERCISE	SETS	REPS ✓	REPS ✓	REPS ✓	REPS ✓
	WEIGHT				
		REPS	REPS	REPS	REPS
	WEIGHT				
		REPS	REPS	REPS	REPS
	WEIGHT				
		REPS	REPS	REPS	REPS
	WEIGHT				
		REPS	REPS	REPS	REPS
	WEIGHT				
		REPS	REPS	REPS	REPS
	WEIGHT				
		REPS	REPS	REPS	REPS
	WEIGHT				
		REPS	REPS	REPS	REPS
	WEIGHT				
		REPS	REPS	REPS	REPS
	WEIGHT				
		REPS	REPS	REPS	REPS
	WEIGHT				

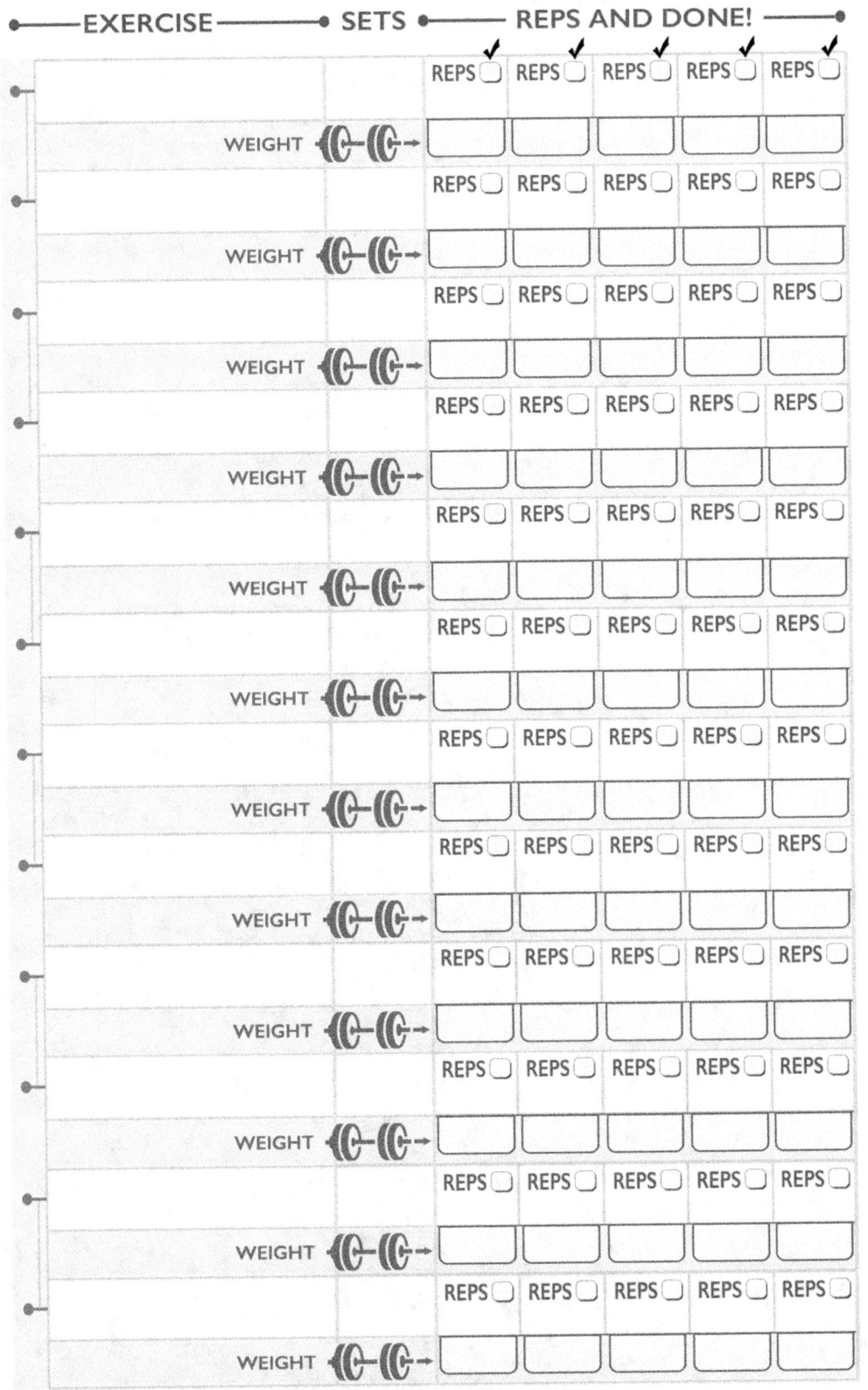

EXERCISE	SETS	REPS AND DONE!			
		REPS ☐	REPS ☐	REPS ☐	REPS ☐
WEIGHT ◖—◖→					
		REPS ☐	REPS ☐	REPS ☐	REPS ☐
WEIGHT ◖—◖→					
		REPS ☐	REPS ☐	REPS ☐	REPS ☐
WEIGHT ◖—◖→					
		REPS ☐	REPS ☐	REPS ☐	REPS ☐
WEIGHT ◖—◖→					
		REPS ☐	REPS ☐	REPS ☐	REPS ☐
WEIGHT ◖—◖→					
		REPS ☐	REPS ☐	REPS ☐	REPS ☐
WEIGHT ◖—◖→					
		REPS ☐	REPS ☐	REPS ☐	REPS ☐
WEIGHT ◖—◖→					
		REPS ☐	REPS ☐	REPS ☐	REPS ☐
WEIGHT ◖—◖→					
		REPS ☐	REPS ☐	REPS ☐	REPS ☐
WEIGHT ◖—◖→					
		REPS ☐	REPS ☐	REPS ☐	REPS ☐
WEIGHT ◖—◖→					

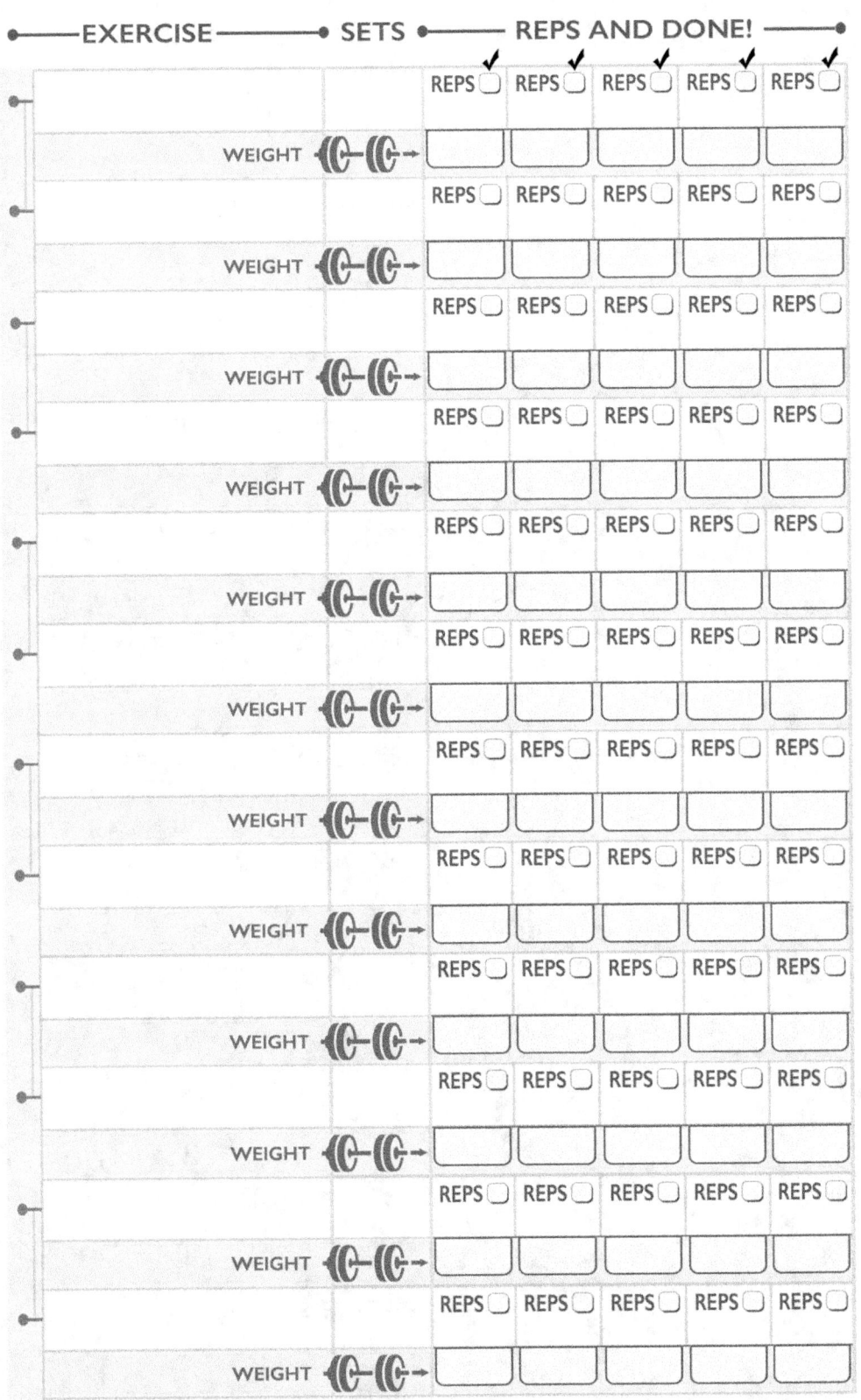

EXERCISE	SETS	REPS	REPS	REPS	REPS
	WEIGHT				
		REPS	REPS	REPS	REPS
	WEIGHT				
		REPS	REPS	REPS	REPS
	WEIGHT				
		REPS	REPS	REPS	REPS
	WEIGHT				
		REPS	REPS	REPS	REPS
	WEIGHT				
		REPS	REPS	REPS	REPS
	WEIGHT				
		REPS	REPS	REPS	REPS
	WEIGHT				
		REPS	REPS	REPS	REPS
	WEIGHT				
		REPS	REPS	REPS	REPS
	WEIGHT				
		REPS	REPS	REPS	REPS
	WEIGHT				
		REPS	REPS	REPS	REPS
	WEIGHT				

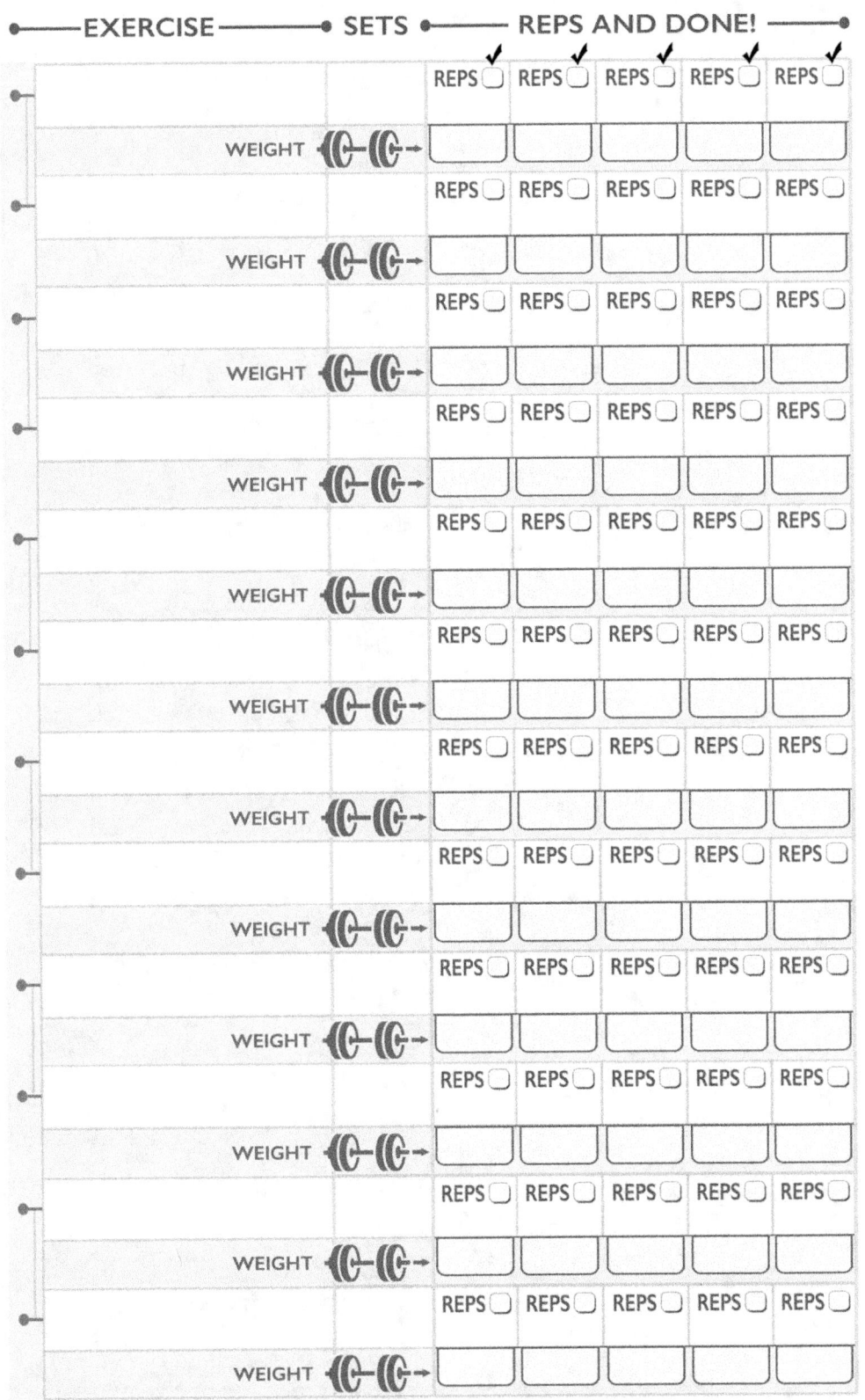

EXERCISE	SETS	REPS ✔	REPS ✔	REPS ✔	REPS ✔
	WEIGHT ◀(●─(●→				
		REPS ☐	REPS ☐	REPS ☐	REPS ☐
	WEIGHT ◀(●─(●→				
		REPS ☐	REPS ☐	REPS ☐	REPS ☐
	WEIGHT ◀(●─(●→				
		REPS ☐	REPS ☐	REPS ☐	REPS ☐
	WEIGHT ◀(●─(●→				
		REPS ☐	REPS ☐	REPS ☐	REPS ☐
	WEIGHT ◀(●─(●→				
		REPS ☐	REPS ☐	REPS ☐	REPS ☐
	WEIGHT ◀(●─(●→				
		REPS ☐	REPS ☐	REPS ☐	REPS ☐
	WEIGHT ◀(●─(●→				
		REPS ☐	REPS ☐	REPS ☐	REPS ☐
	WEIGHT ◀(●─(●→				
		REPS ☐	REPS ☐	REPS ☐	REPS ☐
	WEIGHT ◀(●─(●→				
		REPS ☐	REPS ☐	REPS ☐	REPS ☐
	WEIGHT ◀(●─(●→				
		REPS ☐	REPS ☐	REPS ☐	REPS ☐
	WEIGHT ◀(●─(●→				

EXERCISE	SETS	REPS AND DONE!				
		REPS ☐	REPS ☐	REPS ☐	REPS ☐	REPS ☐
	WEIGHT					
		REPS ☐	REPS ☐	REPS ☐	REPS ☐	REPS ☐
	WEIGHT					
		REPS ☐	REPS ☐	REPS ☐	REPS ☐	REPS ☐
	WEIGHT					
		REPS ☐	REPS ☐	REPS ☐	REPS ☐	REPS ☐
	WEIGHT					
		REPS ☐	REPS ☐	REPS ☐	REPS ☐	REPS ☐
	WEIGHT					
		REPS ☐	REPS ☐	REPS ☐	REPS ☐	REPS ☐
	WEIGHT					
		REPS ☐	REPS ☐	REPS ☐	REPS ☐	REPS ☐
	WEIGHT					
		REPS ☐	REPS ☐	REPS ☐	REPS ☐	REPS ☐
	WEIGHT					
		REPS ☐	REPS ☐	REPS ☐	REPS ☐	REPS ☐
	WEIGHT					
		REPS ☐	REPS ☐	REPS ☐	REPS ☐	REPS ☐
	WEIGHT					

EXERCISE	SETS	REPS AND DONE!			
		REPS ☐	REPS ☐	REPS ☐	REPS ☐
	WEIGHT ◀◉—◉▶				
		REPS ☐	REPS ☐	REPS ☐	REPS ☐
	WEIGHT ◀◉—◉▶				
		REPS ☐	REPS ☐	REPS ☐	REPS ☐
	WEIGHT ◀◉—◉▶				
		REPS ☐	REPS ☐	REPS ☐	REPS ☐
	WEIGHT ◀◉—◉▶				
		REPS ☐	REPS ☐	REPS ☐	REPS ☐
	WEIGHT ◀◉—◉▶				
		REPS ☐	REPS ☐	REPS ☐	REPS ☐
	WEIGHT ◀◉—◉▶				
		REPS ☐	REPS ☐	REPS ☐	REPS ☐
	WEIGHT ◀◉—◉▶				
		REPS ☐	REPS ☐	REPS ☐	REPS ☐
	WEIGHT ◀◉—◉▶				
		REPS ☐	REPS ☐	REPS ☐	REPS ☐
	WEIGHT ◀◉—◉▶				
		REPS ☐	REPS ☐	REPS ☐	REPS ☐
	WEIGHT ◀◉—◉▶				

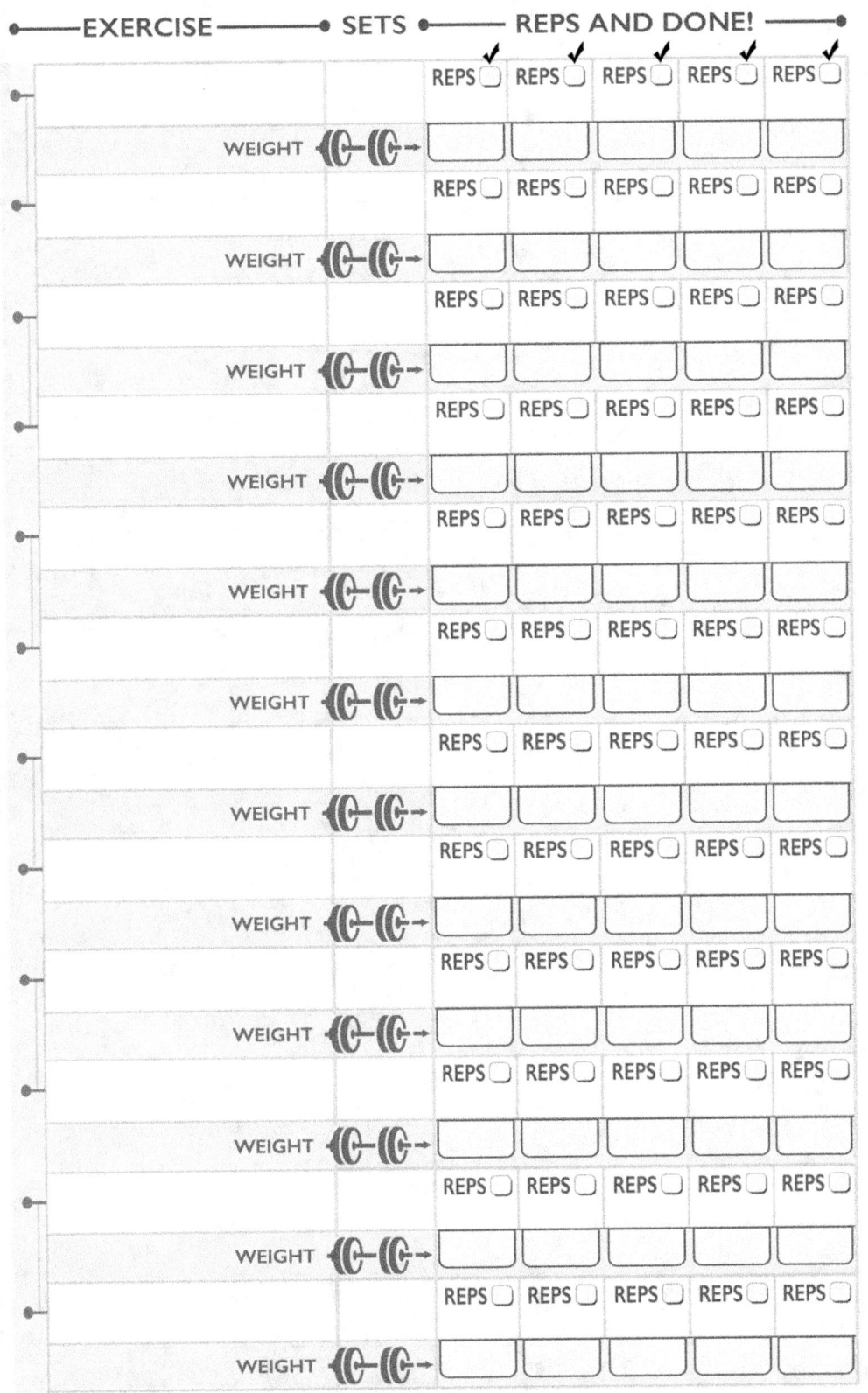

EXERCISE	SETS	REPS AND DONE!			
		REPS ☐	REPS ☐	REPS ☐	REPS ☐
	WEIGHT ◀█─█▶				
		REPS ☐	REPS ☐	REPS ☐	REPS ☐
	WEIGHT ◀█─█▶				
		REPS ☐	REPS ☐	REPS ☐	REPS ☐
	WEIGHT ◀█─█▶				
		REPS ☐	REPS ☐	REPS ☐	REPS ☐
	WEIGHT ◀█─█▶				
		REPS ☐	REPS ☐	REPS ☐	REPS ☐
	WEIGHT ◀█─█▶				
		REPS ☐	REPS ☐	REPS ☐	REPS ☐
	WEIGHT ◀█─█▶				
		REPS ☐	REPS ☐	REPS ☐	REPS ☐
	WEIGHT ◀█─█▶				
		REPS ☐	REPS ☐	REPS ☐	REPS ☐
	WEIGHT ◀█─█▶				
		REPS ☐	REPS ☐	REPS ☐	REPS ☐
	WEIGHT ◀█─█▶				
		REPS ☐	REPS ☐	REPS ☐	REPS ☐
	WEIGHT ◀█─█▶				

EXERCISE	SETS	REPS AND DONE!				
		REPS ☐	REPS ☐	REPS ☐	REPS ☐	REPS ☐
	WEIGHT					
		REPS ☐	REPS ☐	REPS ☐	REPS ☐	REPS ☐
	WEIGHT					
		REPS ☐	REPS ☐	REPS ☐	REPS ☐	REPS ☐
	WEIGHT					
		REPS ☐	REPS ☐	REPS ☐	REPS ☐	REPS ☐
	WEIGHT					
		REPS ☐	REPS ☐	REPS ☐	REPS ☐	REPS ☐
	WEIGHT					
		REPS ☐	REPS ☐	REPS ☐	REPS ☐	REPS ☐
	WEIGHT					
		REPS ☐	REPS ☐	REPS ☐	REPS ☐	REPS ☐
	WEIGHT					
		REPS ☐	REPS ☐	REPS ☐	REPS ☐	REPS ☐
	WEIGHT					
		REPS ☐	REPS ☐	REPS ☐	REPS ☐	REPS ☐
	WEIGHT					
		REPS ☐	REPS ☐	REPS ☐	REPS ☐	REPS ☐
	WEIGHT					

EXERCISE	SETS	REPS AND DONE!			
		REPS ☐	REPS ☐	REPS ☐	REPS ☐
	WEIGHT				
		REPS ☐	REPS ☐	REPS ☐	REPS ☐
	WEIGHT				
		REPS ☐	REPS ☐	REPS ☐	REPS ☐
	WEIGHT				
		REPS ☐	REPS ☐	REPS ☐	REPS ☐
	WEIGHT				
		REPS ☐	REPS ☐	REPS ☐	REPS ☐
	WEIGHT				
		REPS ☐	REPS ☐	REPS ☐	REPS ☐
	WEIGHT				
		REPS ☐	REPS ☐	REPS ☐	REPS ☐
	WEIGHT				
		REPS ☐	REPS ☐	REPS ☐	REPS ☐
	WEIGHT				
		REPS ☐	REPS ☐	REPS ☐	REPS ☐
	WEIGHT				
		REPS ☐	REPS ☐	REPS ☐	REPS ☐
	WEIGHT				

EXERCISE	SETS	REPS AND DONE!
		REPS ☑ REPS ☑ REPS ☑ REPS ☑ REPS ☑
WEIGHT		REPS ☐ REPS ☐ REPS ☐ REPS ☐ REPS ☐
WEIGHT		REPS ☐ REPS ☐ REPS ☐ REPS ☐ REPS ☐
WEIGHT		REPS ☐ REPS ☐ REPS ☐ REPS ☐ REPS ☐
WEIGHT		REPS ☐ REPS ☐ REPS ☐ REPS ☐ REPS ☐
WEIGHT		REPS ☐ REPS ☐ REPS ☐ REPS ☐ REPS ☐
WEIGHT		REPS ☐ REPS ☐ REPS ☐ REPS ☐ REPS ☐
WEIGHT		REPS ☐ REPS ☐ REPS ☐ REPS ☐ REPS ☐
WEIGHT		REPS ☐ REPS ☐ REPS ☐ REPS ☐ REPS ☐
WEIGHT		REPS ☐ REPS ☐ REPS ☐ REPS ☐ REPS ☐
WEIGHT		REPS ☐ REPS ☐ REPS ☐ REPS ☐ REPS ☐
WEIGHT